Handbook of Obesity Intervention for the Lifespan

Larry C. James · John C. Linton
Editors

Handbook of Obesity Intervention for the Lifespan

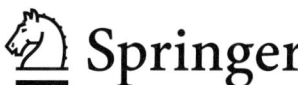 Springer

Editors

Larry C. James
Wright State University
Dayton, Ohio, USA
Larry.James@US.Army.Mil

John C. Linton
West Virginia University School
of Medicine, Charleston
West Virginia, USA
jlinton@hsc.wvu.edu

ISBN: 978-0-387-78304-8   e-ISBN: 978-0-387-78305-5
DOI 10.1007/978-0-387-78305-5

Library of Congress Control Number: 2008938228

Printed on acid-free paper

springer.com

To the lovely and talented ladies in my life, Devon and Lesley, daughters who would make any father proud, Alina Margaret, whose youthful eyes are filled with wonder, and to my wife Shareen, who is simply the best, this book is dedicated with affection and gratitude.

JCL

This book is dedicated to the memory of my mother Mary Harden-James.

LCJ

Contents

Part III   Treatment Resources for Providers

Contributors

Brook L. Barbera, MA
Pennington Biomedical Research Center, Louisiana State University System, Baton Rouge, LA, USA

E. McCrea Fry, RN, BSN
Department of Pediatrics, UAMS College of Medicine, Arkansas Children's Hospital, Little Rock, AR, USA, wardbegnochewendyl@uams.edu

Larry C. James, PhD, ABPP
School of Professional Psychology, Wright State University, 3640 Colonel Glenn Highway, Dayton, OH, USA, Larry.James@Wright.Edu

Reginald Labossiere, MD, CNSP
Donald W. Reynolds Department of Geriatric Medicine, University of Oklahoma Health Science Center and VA Medical Center, Oklahoma City, OK, USA

John C. Linton, PhD, ABPP
Department of Behavioral Medicine and Psychiatry, West Virginia University School of Medicine, Charleston, WV, USA

Vicki McNeill, PT, DPT
Department of Pediatrics, UAMS College of Medicine, Arkansas Children's Hospital, Little Rock, AR, USA

Duncan C. Meyers, MA
Department of Psychology, Barnwell College, University of South Carolina, Columbia, SC, USA

Valerie H. Myers, PhD
Pennington Biomedical Research Center, Louisiana State University System, Baton Rouge, LA, USA, valerie.myers@pbrc.edu

Tracie L. Pasold, PhD
Department of Pediatrics, UAMS College of Medicine, Arkansas Children's Hospital, Little Rock, AR, USA

K. Deane Peck, MS, RD, LDN
Department of Pediatrics, UAMS College of Medicine, Arkansas Children's Hospital, Little Rock, AR, USA

Samiya Razzaq, MD, FAAP
Department of Pediatrics, UAMS College of Medicine, Arkansas Children's Hospital,
Little Rock, AR, USA

Karen M. Ross, MD
*Donald W. Reynolds Department of Geriatric Medicine, University of Oklahoma Health
Sciences Center, Oklahoma City, OK, USA*

Robert B. Shin, MD, FACS
CAMC Weight Loss Center, Charleston Area Medical Center, Charleston, WV, USA

Stephen B. Sondike, MD
Department of Pediatrics, West Virginia University School of Medicine, Adolescent
Medicine, Charleston Area Medical Center, Charleston, WA, USA,
ssondike@hsc.wvu.edu

Kristen H. Sorocco, PhD
*Donald W. Reynolds Department of Geriatric Medicine, University of Oklahoma Health
Sciences Center and VA Medical Center, Oklahoma City, OK, USA,*
Kristen-sorocco@ouhsc.edu

Mark Verschell, PsyD
Health Psychology Service, *Department of Psychology,* Tripler Army Medical Center,
Honolulu, HI, USA, mark.verschell@us.army.mil

Wendy L. Ward-Begnoche, PhD
Department of Pediatrics, UAMS College of Medicine, Arkansas Children's Hospital,
Little Rock, AR, USA

Dawn K. Wilson, PhD
*Department of Psychology, Barnwell College, University of South Carolina, Columbia, SC,
USA,* wilsondk@mailbox.sc.edu

K. Beth Yano, PhD
Child Psychology Service, Department of Psychology, Tripler Army Medical Center,
Honolulu, HI, USA, kbethyano@hawaii.rr.com

Karen L. Young, MD, FAAP
Department of Pediatrics, UAMS College of Medicine, Arkansas Children's Hospital,
Little Rock, AR, USA

Part I
Child and Adolescent Obesity Applications

Introduction

Larry C. James and John C. Linton

Weight problems and obesity in America have continued to accelerate at an unprecedented rate. From childhood through adulthood to old age, Americans are shouldering the burden of obesity and its co-morbid disorders. Weight problems are created by a complicated array of factors that many struggle with on a daily basis. The intricate combination of a sedentary lifestyle, physical illness, psychological issues, genetics, food selection, and environmental forces makes long-term weight loss difficult to achieve. For example, adults and seniors have become less active, and unlike school systems years ago, many public schools no longer offer physical education programs, while young people more readily opt for long stretches of time before a television screen, rather than engaging in active play. In the United States, inactive computer gaming now substitutes for the jump ropes and ball fields of the past.

What causes obesity, and is it mostly environmental or genetic? Do the causes vary in their influence over the life of an individual patient? Are there key components to any successful weight loss program, and can obesity be effectively treated over the lifespan? Are surgical interventions to be the cure of the future for this obesity crisis?

These are but a few questions *Treating Obesity Across the Lifespan* addresses in a practical style. Few books on obesity serve as a one-source reference on this topic, since most are confined to teenage or adult weight problems, whereas this book examines obesity over the lifetimes of patients.

The authors are a collection of scientists and practitioners from throughout the United States, who offer an applied handbook for the healthcare provider in the clinical setting. Unlike most research books, this also provides the reader with useful suggestions for treating weight problems and obesity in their patients.

This handbook began as an obesity project in Hawaii, when the first author began a multi-disciplinary treatment program for adults in 1995. The success of the program led to the creation of a similar program for youth as well as older adults. Both of the programs were extremely successful, and the authors sought to capture the nucleus of these and similar efforts in a single handbook reference for the clinician.

Part I of the book is devoted to the understanding and treatment of childhood and adolescent obesity. Part II focuses exclusively on obesity treatment applications for the adult and elderly populations. Part III provides a list of resources that might be of assistance to clinicians treating patients with weight problems. This handbook offers empirically based clinical interventions that consider a wide variety of patient variables.

L.C. James (✉)
School of Professional Psychology, Wright State University, 3640 Colonel Glenn Highway, Dayton, OH, USA
e-mail: Larry.James@Wright.Edu

L.C. James, J.C. Linton (eds.), *Handbook of Obesity Intervention for the Lifespan*, DOI 10.1007/978-0-387-78305-5_1, © Springer Science+Business Media, LLC 2009

Topics range from in-depth examination of core literature to specific recommendations for the 10 steps to a healthy lifestyle, regardless of one's age.

We have found that obesity is best conceptualized as a disease that requires treatment across the life of the patient. Accordingly, we have organized a clinical handbook that is rare in the field, one that provides assessment and treatment options for clinicians who work with obese patients, young or old.

Chapter 1
Childhood Obesity Treatment Literature Review

Wendy L. Ward-Begnoche, Tracie L. Pasold, Vicki McNeill, K. Deane Peck, Samiya Razzaq, E. McCrea Fry, and Karen L. Young

Childhood obesity is an urgent problem deserving clinical attention and community resources. There are several key treatment concepts that are unique to the treatment of children: (1) treatment must be family centered, (2) treatment must be developmentally appropriate, (3) weight goals are complicated in growing children, and (4) malnutrition must be addressed and good nutrition continued during treatment to maintain normal linear growth and health (Barlow & Dietz, 1998; American Academy of Pediatrics, 2003; Expert Committee, 2007). Furthermore, complications of obesity can be both medical and psychological, which must be uncovered and treated in order to have optimal health and successful weight management. Common medical problems encountered involve the cardiovascular and respiratory systems (Calderon, Yucha, & Schaffer, 2005; Gidding et al., 2004), chronic pain (Marcus, 2004), insulin resistance (Young-Hyman, Schlundt, Herman, De Luca, & Counts, 2001), and other endocrine disorders (Quattrin, Liu, Shaw, Shine, & Chiang, 2005). They are at risk of developing type 2 diabetes, which causes an increase in adult mortality and morbidity rates (Must & Strauss, 1999). They are also at risk of developing multiple psychiatric and psychological disorders such as depression, anxiety, and low self-esteem (Zametkin, Zoon, Klein, & Munson, 2004). Finally, as obese children become adults, they are likely to remain obese and are at risk of developing many weight-related co-morbidities, which cause an increase in adult mortality and morbidity rates (Must & Strauss, 1999).

Evidence-based treatment of overweight and obese children incorporates a multidisciplinary approach, including medical treatment, nutrition education, physical activity education, family involvement, and behavior modification (Jefferson, 2005; Zametkin et al., 2004; AAP, 2003; Expert Committee, 2007). Recommendations from health-care providers should address the following areas: medical care, food choices and eating patterns, physical activity choices and patterns, family strengths and challenges (family eating and activity patterns, parenting skills, parent perceptions of weight and health status), personal strengths and challenges (motivation, disordered eating patterns, psychological state), and environmental and community access/support. Individualized goal setting is critical and must take into account all of these factors.

W.L. Ward-Begnoche (✉)

Department of Pediatrics, UAMS College of Medicine, Arkansas Children's Hospital, Little Rock, AR, 72202-3591, USA

e-mail: wardbegnochewendyl@uams.edu

L.C. James, J.C. Linton (eds.), *Handbook of Obesity Intervention for the Lifespan*,
DOI 10.1007/978-0-387-78305-5_2, © Springer Science+Business Media, LLC 2009

Medical Evaluation and Treatment of Children

Abnormal weight gain is defined as an upward crossing of percentiles on the body mass index (BMI) portion of the growth chart for children and adolescents between 2 and 19 years. For babies and toddlers between birth and 2 years, BMI is not utilized. Instead, the weight/length chart is used for those under 2 years. Any child noted to have abnormal weight gain should have a detailed evaluation to determine the underlying etiology for the abnormal weight gain (AAP, 2003). Medical providers should assess weight status by calculating and plotting BMI. They should also assess diet and exercise patterns in all children and adolescents yearly. Children or adolescents found to be either overweight (BMI between the 85th and 95th percentiles for age and gender) or obese (BMI $\geq$ 95th percentile for age and gender), or babies under 2 years with weight/length $\geq$ 95th percentile, should have focused family histories, physical examinations, and laboratory studies done in addition to specific intervention (AAP, 2003).

Evidence-based treatment of overweight youth now is a staged protocol, as recommended by the Expert Committee on the Assessment, Prevention and Treatment of Child and Adolescent Overweight and Obesity, released on June 8, 2007. This committee, made up of representatives from 15 health professional organizations, was convened by the American Medical Association (AMA). The first two stages can be implemented by the primary care physician or allied health-care provider who has some training in pediatric weight management/behavioral counseling. At these stages the provider counsels the family to implement healthy lifestyle changes in diet and physical activity and to decrease sedentary activities, with a goal to maintain the weight while age and height increase. The level of intervention becomes more intensified if the patient does not respond at the first two stages of treatment.

Child and Family Goals: Stage 1

- Five or more fruits and vegetables/day
- Two or less hours of screen time/day
- No TV in bedroom
- One hour or more of physical activity
- No sugar-sweetened beverages
- Eat breakfast daily
- Limit meals eaten out
- Family meals 5-6 times/week
- Allow the child to learn to self-regulate food intake
- Try to maintain weight
- If no improvement in BMI in 3-6, advance to Stage 2

Source: Spear B., Barlow S., Ervin C., Ludwig D., Saelens B., Schetzine K., Taveras E. (2007). Recommendations for Treatment of Child and Adolescent Overweight and Obesity, Pediatrics, 120, S254–288.

At stage three, it is recommended that a comprehensive multidisciplinary intervention is instituted by a specialty obesity care team. At stages three and four, the multidisciplinary team should employ the following activities: structured behavior management program with training of primary caregivers and food and activity monitoring. The multidisciplinary team should address meal replacement, very low calorie diet, medication, and surgery as indicated (Expert Committee, 2007).

Structured Weight Management: Stage 2

- Balanced macro-nutrient diet, with low amounts of energy-dense foods
- Structured daily meals and snacks
- Screen time 1 hour or less/day

- Monitoring logs (screen time, physical activity, food intake) checked by provider
- Weight goal of maintenance or loss not to exceed 1 lb/mo in ages 2-11 or 2 lb/wk in teens

Comprehensive Multidisciplinary Protocol: Stage 3

- Should optimally be referred to a multidisciplinary obesity care team
- Eating and activity goals are the same as in Stage 2
- Should also include a structured behavior modification program

- Involve primary caregivers and family in training for behavior modification
- Weight goals may be weight maintenance, or no more than 1 lb/mo in 2-5 years or 2 lb/wk in older children and teens

Tertiary Care Protocol: Stage 4

- Referral to pediatric tertiary weight management center
- Continued diet and activity counseling

- Consideration of such additions as meal replacement, very-low-calorie diet, medication, and surgery

Source: Spear B., Barlow S., Ervin C., Ludwig D., Saelens B., Schetzine K., Taveras E. (2007). Recommendations for Treatment of Child and Adolescent Overweight and Obesity, Pediatrics, 120, S254–288.

Any child examined by their physician and noted to have abnormal weight gain should have a detailed evaluation to determine the underlying etiology (AAP, 2003). It is important to screen for obesity-related co-morbidities such as hypertension, dyslipidemia, hyperinsulinemia, impaired glucose tolerance, and obstructive sleep apnea (AAP, 2003). This is particularly important if the patient is currently symptomatic or has a personal or family history of the disease.

Cardiovascular Conditions

In the Bogalusa Heart study, more than 60% of obese children had at least one risk factor for cardiovascular disease (Dietz and Robinson, 2005). Metabolic syndrome in children has been found to be a sensitive predictor of future cardiovascular disease (Litwin et al., 2007). Hypertension is a common problem in overweight individuals. All children should have their blood pressure monitored if they have an elevated BMI. It is important to use the proper method and equipment. The latest blood pressure charts for the pediatric age group use age, sex, and height percentile to determine norms (National High Blood Pressure Education Program, 2004). A low-salt, low-fat diet along with a regular exercise program is initiated when the blood pressure elevation is first detected. Urinalysis, BUN, and creatinine should be checked. If persistently elevated at least three times on different visits, recommendations are to typically follow a no-added-salt, low-fat, no-concentrated-sweets diet and have regular exercise. If the blood pressure does not normalize, medication management should be considered.

Overweight children are identified as being particularly at high risk for cardiovascular disease if there is at least one family member with a history of cardiovascular disease, especially a first-degree relative. Fatty streaks have been found in the arteries of adolescents as young as 13 years of age (Strong, Malcom, Newman, & Oalmann, 1992). A lipid panel should be ordered to assess for dyslipidemia. If abnormal, defined as elevated total cholesterol, elevated LDL cholesterol, elevated triglycerides, or decreased HDL cholesterol, therapeutic lifestyle and dietary modifications should be initiated. Treatment consists of low-cholesterol and/or low-fat diet, combined with regular physical activity for at least 3–6 months. If the child is at least 9 years old and has not responded to dietary intervention, then adding a statin medication is considered.

Insulin Resistance–Associated Conditions

There are several obesity-related conditions due to insulin resistance. These include conditions that directly lead to type 2 diabetes: hyperinsulinism, impaired fasting glucose, and also such diverse sounding conditions as non-alcoholic fatty liver disease and polycystic ovarian syndrome. One study evaluated 103 obese (BMI $\geq$ 95th percentile) children and adolescents 2–18 years of age. Abnormal glucose homeostasis was identified in 46% (hyperinsulinism in 40%, impaired fasting glucose in 0.8%, and impaired glucose tolerance in 11%) (Vincer, Segal, Lichtarowicz-Krynska, & Hindmarsh, 2005). Insulin resistance is likely to be present if the child has acanthosis nigricans on physical examination. If there is a family history of diabetes or the child is of Hispanic or African-American background, the risk is even higher. Having a high insulin level causes abnormal hunger, perpetuating the cycle of abnormal eating behaviors. Screening for diseases related to insulin resistance may help families understand the seriousness of their child's obesity-related disease and increase their compliance with the dietary treatment. To help the child who has insulin resistance, the health providers must get the child's insulin level down (See Nutrition Section). If insulin resistance can be reversed, the child's acanthosis nigricans will lighten and may even disappear, the insulin level and hunger will normalize, and the risk for diabetes will drop.

Respiratory Conditions

Obstructive sleep apnea can occur throughout childhood. Screen for this condition by asking if the child has sleep problems with snoring, gasping, apnea greater than 15 s, disrupted sleep, daytime drowsiness, declining school performance, irritability, or early morning headaches. If there are concerns, referral and a sleep study should be considered and appropriate treatment instituted. This is one condition where rapid weight loss in the morbidly obese child may need to be considered because sleep apnea carries significant morbidity and mortality and the only other treatments available are life altering and invasive (Barlow and Dietz, 1998). These include the use of BIPAP/CPAP machines at night or surgical interventions with an adenotonsillectomy (Schwimmer et al., 2003), an uvulopalatoplasty, or, as a last resort, a tracheostomy. Consider obtaining an EKG and a chest x-ray on any child with a BMI > 40 or long-standing untreated sleep apnea to screen for heart failure.

Childhood obesity is associated with the development of asthma, but the mechanisms underlying this relationship have not yet been delineated. Abnormal weight gain can precede the development of asthma, as shown in a number of prospective studies. Furthermore, weight reduction among asthmatic patients can result in improvements of lung function (Schaub & von Mutius, 2005). The differential diagnosis of the dyspneic patient can be tricky. The patient with asthma will likely cough at night or with exercise; the patient with obesity hypoventilation syndrome or sleep apnea may have sonorous respirations even while awake and be tired and lethargic; the patient who is just sedentary and out of shape will have dyspnea only with exercise and have difficulty keeping up with peers.

Musculoskeletal Conditions

Overweight children can experience various musculoskeletal problems because of the excess weight on their joints. Some of these problems include flat feet, fractures, joint pain especially in the knee, and lower extremity malalignment, all of which can limit mobility and contribute to additional weight gain because the children cannot participate in activity without pain.

Two specific musculoskeletal problems related to overweight children are Blount's disease and slipped capital femoral epiphysis (SCFE). These conditions may significantly limit the child's participation in physical activity and result in lifelong problems if not identified and treated properly. Blount's disease is a growth disorder of the tibia, resulting in bowing. Obesity and early walking exaggerate the bowing. Unless diagnosed and treated early, the condition progressively worsens. Treatment may include bracing for children between the ages of 2 and 5 years and/or later surgery (Tachdijian, 2002). SCFE occurs when shearing and weakening of the femoral epiphysis cause the femoral capital epiphysis to displace. Obesity is a risk factor for developing SCFE because of the increased shearing forces. Treatment usually involves surgical pinning (Tachdijian, 2002).

Weight Goals

The first weight goal should always be to stop rapid, abnormal weight gain, if present. This can be achieved by uncovering eating behaviors such as consuming large portions, multiple seconds, emotional eating, nocturnal eating, skipping meals, and binge eating, and by providing guidance to the parent and child in slowing down and changing these eating behaviors (Young, 2005).

Maintenance of the current weight is appropriate for most overweight and obese children and adolescents who still have height growth left (Dietz and Robinson, 2005). It is also the first step for those who will ultimately need to begin to lose weight. Weight should be monitored regularly, and if weight is increasing, decrease caloric intake and/or increase physical activity. Maintain the weight until the BMI is less than 85th percentile. (Spear et al, 2007)

Weight loss is imperative for those obese children and adolescents who have life-threatening co-morbid conditions, obesity hypoventilation syndrome, a BMI so elevated that they weigh more than is normal for their ultimate adult height, and for obese adolescents with closed growth plates.

Nutrition Assessment and Treatment

Nutritional assessment involves the gathering of information about characteristics of daily living that include the following: eating and drinking habits/patterns, exercise and activity habits, weight and dieting history, food allergies, medical history, nutrition knowledge, and social interactions. The quality of the dietary intake can be assessed using a 3–7 day dietary recall and/or 24-hours dietary recall. Any dietary history of food and beverage intake should include the following: number of meals and snacks eaten daily, types of meals and snacks eaten, amounts of foods and beverages consumed, time that the meals and snacks are eaten, number of servings from each of the food groups in the past 7 days, identifiable food problem behaviors (e.g., where, when, how, and why children are eating), and the persons and places involved in buying, preparing, and serving meals and snacks. The family unit should be assessed and utilized in the evaluation and encouraged to participate in the treatment plan along with the individual child for optimal care (Vila et al., 2004). Dietitians can then identify areas of nutritional and lifestyle changes that need to take place in order to help the patient.

Nutritional recommendations must take into account the family situation. Identifying maladaptive eating patterns in family members can provide clues as to the etiology of patients' eating patterns. Furthermore, uncovering reasons for the entire family's lack of support of nutritional changes and engaging all family members (siblings, parents, grandparents, and anyone involved regularly with the child) is absolutely critical to creating positive change in the child's eating behaviors (Vila et al., 2004).

The child's and the caregiver's level of knowledge about nutritional concepts must be assessed. Often individuals are misinformed about important nutritional concepts, including *portion size, balanced meal, metabolism, healthy eating,* and *low fat*. Using nutrition and activity terminology with patients does not guarantee good communication or goal achievement. Omar, Coleman, and Hoerr (2001) reported that caregivers, in general, relied on other family members as the source of most nutrition information whether the information was accurate or not. The disparity among caregivers opens avenues for educating families, and in some cases, must include the extended family. Miscommunications and misunderstandings of the meanings of commonly used terms can be avoided with a careful review of key concepts and/or educational handouts (Ward-Begnoche & Gance-Cleveland, 2005).

After the initial assessment of the nutritional intake is done and the general knowledge of key concepts in nutrition is assessed, specific nutrition recommendations must be tailored to the individual patient. Patients with co-morbid medical conditions should have nutritional recommendations tailored to their specific needs. A specific diet addressing the patient's unique nutritional patterns and/or medical co-morbidities is needed—low sodium, low cholesterol, low sugar or less sugary drinks, more fruits/vegetables, among others. Goals should be specific and clear. Vitamin D supplementation and multivitamins are often recommended due to the limited intake of dairy products and low intake of nutrient-dense foods.

If insulin resistance is diagnosed, portion control along with other nutritional changes such as having routine meals and snacks, keeping 2–4 h between the meals and the snacks, using portion sizes that are age specific for all foods and beverages, and using high-fiber foods along with other nutrient-dense foods can aid in lowering the insulin level. Reducing all concentrated sweets, such as sugar-sweetened beverages, cookies, and cakes, and watching portion sizes on complex carbohydrates, such as white flour products (e.g., bread, potatoes, rice, pastas, and corn,) are also critical. In addition, substituting whole grain carbohydrates for white flour products will cause a more gradual rise in insulin. This can help stabilize the secretion of insulin and reduce the intense hunger typical of elevated serum insulin levels. Pairing protein-dense food with high-fiber complex carbohydrate at meals and snacks along with unlimited amounts of non-starch vegetables can help produce satiety. High-protein/low-carbohydrate diets or any other nutritional plan that involves unbalanced intake are not recommended.

Commonly identified barriers to change in family lifestyles are as follows: finding low-cost healthy meals, modifying family cooking strategies, budgeting distribution of food throughout the month, focusing on changes in intake patterns, reducing foods of minimal nutritional value, and school-based education programs (Cawley, 2006).

Even after learning about food types, serving sizes, and balancing meals, some are still unable to make appropriate nutritional choices because of the family's financial situation. Patients and their families need education on how to buy healthy foods on a limited income. For others, learning how to budget and distribute food throughout the month is important. It is always a good idea to purchase fresh fruits and vegetables in season and on sale. Most grocery stores will always have fresh, frozen, or canned fruits and vegetables on sale. Shopping food circulars and using coupons along with other aids such as food stamps and vouchers can help with healthier food choices. Intervention efforts to overcome obstacles should focus on structured family planning. Advocating for laws, school policies, and social service changes that affect the cost of food and access to healthy foods can influence children in a positive way.

Nutritional intake should be a health-related goal separate from weight loss or weight maintenance. It is critical to understand that positive changes in the child's dietary intake and/or nutrient status will improve their health even in the absence of weight loss (better self-esteem, disease prevention, etc.) (American Dietetic Association, 2006).

Physical Fitness Assessment and Treatment

While nutritional factors relate to the rise in obesity, a general decline in the physical activity of children is also to blame. Excessive screen time has been correlated with weight gain and sedentary behavior (Andersen, Crespo, Bartlett, Cheskin, & Pratt, 1988; Faith et al., 2001). Data from the 1988–1994 National Health and Nutrition Examination Survey indicated that 26% of children (33% of Mexican American and 43% of non-Hispanic black children) watched at least 4 h of television per day. These same children were also less likely to participate in physical activity (Anderson et al., 1998). Overweight parents are associated with decreased physical activity in their children (Sallis, Prochaska, & Taylor, 2000; Treuth, Butte, Adolph, & Puyau, 2004). In addition, there may be barriers that prevent a child's participation in physical activity, including financial restrictions and facility accessibility.

In a study involving 20 large U.S. cities, mothers' perceptions of neighborhood safety were related to their children's TV viewing time (Burdette & Whitaker, 2005).

Exercise Prescriptions

In an effort to address the issue of increased sedentary behavior and help prevent the onset of overweight in children, the American Academy of Pediatrics (AAP) has recommended 2 h or less of total screen time (which includes TV viewing, computer use, and video games) daily. Likewise, the AAP recommends children should be encouraged to be active and engaged in play for a minimum of 1 h daily to achieve the recommended levels of physical activity. However, telling them simply to move is often not enough. Some children and families require specific instructions. Fulton, Garg, Galuska, Rattay, and Caspersen (2004) summarized in their article recommendations from 10 organizations specializing in physical fitness or physical activity. These authors found that about half of the recommendations targeted both children and adolescents, and that of the four components of physical activity—frequency, duration, intensity, and type; most recommendations included at least three. Frequency recommendations ranged from three to five or more times per week to daily. Generally, the activity intensity was recommended as moderate or vigorous. Duration varied from 20 min of vigorous physical activity to 60 min of moderate physical activity. Benefits are increased when the activity is performed with greater intensity such as running instead of walking. Sothern and colleagues (1999) recommend physical exercise that is both structured and progressive.

Key physical activity concepts are also often misunderstood by patients, for example, *screen time, moderate intensity, cardiovascular fitness, flexibility, strength training,* and *low impact.* It is critical for providers to review these concepts with patients in detail and/or use explanatory handouts to avoid misunderstanding and miscommunication (Ward-Begnoche & Gance-Cleveland, 2005).

The type of activity chosen for overweight children should be those that are fun and age appropriate. For example, the AAP suggests that preschool children (aged 4–6 years) should be encouraged to engage in free play, with the emphasis on fun, exploration, and experimentation including both structured and unstructured play. Examples of activities that would satisfy these requirements include the following: running while playing games such as chase, "freeze tag," jumping as in hopscotch, climbing on playground equipment, and tumbling. For the elementary school age child (6–9 years), free play with more sophisticated movement patterns is encouraged. Activities such as bicycling, swimming, jumping rope, walking, dancing, and beginner organized sports would be good choices. For the middle-school child (10–12 years), the AAP recommends focusing on enjoyment in activity but increasing focus on tactics and strategy of sports. Clinicians and parents both should recognize that a gradual increase in these parameters may be necessary for a child that is not accustomed to activity. Efforts should be made to decrease the screen time while increasing the physical activity.

Individualizing the plan for some children may be necessary as some will perform best with structured activities such as sports or classes, while others may prefer to be active with family or a friend or alone. Organized sports are useful methods to provide activity on a regular and consistent basis, but knowing the child and their preferences is important in helping them succeed. Seasonal variations in activity are common but should not be used as excuses to be inactive. Indoor activities and facilities that provide protection from harsh temperatures should be substituted in these instances or adjustments made to one's schedule to avoid extreme temperatures. Clinicians can assist the families in problem solving and avoiding barriers from becoming obstacles by providing them with handouts that list no-cost or low-cost options appropriate for different settings (in house, out of house, with others, solitary, etc.) and different weather conditions (Ward-Begnoche & Gance-Cleveland, 2005). Ask the child to review this list or compile their own list of all the physical activities they enjoy (Sallis, Prochaska, &Taylor 2000) plus add activities that they might like to try. Encouraging families to participate in physical activity with their children reinforces the behavior change and models healthy exercise habits. Keep in mind that, sometimes, several short bursts of physical activity are more logistically possible than a longer bout, and they may be more reinforcing for children and adolescents (Epstein et al., 2001). Stefan, Hopman, and Smythe (2005) reported that children who were exercise intolerant or activity restricted due to a medical condition experienced larger increases in BMI and ranked higher in their BMI percentile than children with neither condition. Medical conditions can often have a strong impact on physical activity recommendations. For instance, children with chronic joint pain often avoid physical activity or find it difficult to engage in such activity. Children and their parents should seek alternative environments or activities to substitute for an activity that is perceived as aggravating. Providing alternative activities that help lessen weight bearing such as swimming or bicycling can be effective while maintaining some physical activity. Families will need to be educated on how to set reasonable goals for physical activity; how to avoid boredom by changing the activity or setting regularly; to understand that some exercise is better than nothing on days when the goal cannot be achieved; and finally how to treat common aches and pains associated with overuse.

Asthmatic reactions during exercise can also complicate activity recommendations. For example, children with asthma often experience exercise-induced asthma (EIA) which, without proper instruction on how to manage, can result in a decrease in activity. Short bursts of activity generally do not produce EIA symptoms; likewise, swimming seldom causes EIA. Pre-medicating with a prescribed inhaler 15–30 min before exercise can prevent an attack. It is important to note that a recent study showed that there was no correlation between asthma severity and aerobic fitness (Pianosi & Davis, 2004). Only perceived competence at physical activity was found to have a significant correlation with aerobic fitness, so the exercise intolerance often reported by overweight asthmatic patients may be more due to perceived lower competence at physical activities than actual asthmatic reactions. Given the wide range of medical co-morbidities associated with childhood obesity (see medical assessment section), these conditions must be taken into account when designing an individualized physical activity plan.

Familial Influence on Treatment

Eating and activity behaviors are modeled for children by parents. The family can influence successful weight reduction in multiple ways, including parental modeling of a healthy lifestyle, providing a supportive atmosphere, and reducing family stressors. If that modeling shows poor nutritional choices and a sedentary lifestyle, children will mimic these behaviors. In fact, parent self-report of activity accounted for some of the variance in overweight children's physical activity (Epstein, Vito, & Anderson, 1996). Parental food choice and purchasing behaviors may influence how children purchase both healthy and unhealthy foods (Epstein, Dearing, Handley, Roemmich, & Paluch, 2006), and family mealtimes in adolescence are associated with more positive dietary choices and healthy behaviors (Cason, 2006). In addition, parental weight status for both mothers and fathers is associated with the weight status of their children (Baughcum, Chamberlin, Deeks, Powers, & Whitaker, 2000; Golan, Weizman, & Fainaru, 1999; Strauss & Knight, 1999), and parent overweight status is associated with the child's physical activity level (Sallis et al., 2000; Treuth et al., 2004).

Parental disciplinary strategies also have an important impact on children's behavior (Ogden, Reynolds, & Smith, 2006). An authoritarian approach to parenting often results in a battle of wills with children, which can create standoffs (e.g., when children are ordered to sit at the table for hours in attempts to force them to try fruits and vegetables or other new items [Omar et al., 2001]). In fact, authoritarian parenting was associated with the highest risk of overweight among young children (Rhee, Lumeng, Appugliese, Kaciroti, & Bradley, 2006). However, parental control of nutritional intake and structured planning regarding healthy behaviors is not always negative (Chen & Kennedy, 2004).

Parental views of their children's weight also have an important role in the treatment. Parents often do not see their children as overweight even when they are, and some parents may view heavy children as being healthy and as a sign of successful parenting (Adams, Quinn, & Prince, 2005; Baughcum et al., 2000). They may use terms such as "big-boned" or "solid" rather than "overweight" when describing their children. Mothers only believe their child has developed a problem with obesity when they begin to suffer the effects of teasing or physical limitations (Jain et al., 2001). Furthermore, parents often attribute overweight to an inherited difficulty, citing multiple overweight family members, while disregarding the influence of the family environment on weight status (Faulkner, 2002).

Persuading parents to be concerned is critical, especially because parental concern about weight is an important predictor of change in total fat mass over time, at least in Caucasian children (Jain et al., 2001). Parents are more likely to be motivated to change when they view their child's weight as a health problem (Rhee, DeLago, Arscott-Mills, Mehta, & Davis, 2005).

It becomes obvious that family assessment and involvement in the treatment plan is crucial (Dietz, 1983; Epstein, Valoski, Wing, & McCurley, 1994; Vila et al., 2004). Research suggests that parental behaviors regarding nutritional diet and physical activity affect a child's attitude toward the recommended lifestyle changes (Levine, Ringham, Kalarchian, Wisniewski, & Marcus, 2001; Zametkin et al., 2004). In fact, parent changes in BMI have been found to predict child changes in BMI for overweight youth (Wrotniak, Epstein, Paluch, & Roemmich, 2004). As noted earlier, parenting style and disciplinary strategies can serve as barriers. Family discussions are a necessary component in the process of informing and engaging family members in assessment and behavioral change processes, uncovering erroneous belief systems, identifying family dynamics that may affect treatment, and assessing parenting skills. It is important to facilitate the parents' understanding of how their roles in addressing nutrition and physical activity need to evolve as their children move through different developmental periods (Lindsay, Sussner, Kim, & Gortmaker, 2006), suggesting the importance of a flexible parenting style that evolves as the child ages.

Personal Influences on Treatment

Overweight children have a larger number of psychosocial problems than normal-weight children (Young-Hyman, Schlundt, Herman-Wenderoth, & Bozylinski, 2003). A review of the past 10 years of published research on the psychiatric aspects of pediatric obesity shows increased rates of depression, anxiety, and self-esteem (Zametkin et al., 2004), which can be significant barriers to change in overweight youths (Strauss, 2000). Emotional difficulties can cause an increase in distress that contributes to binging and overeating (Zametkin et al., 2004), limit physical activity, and impair motivation to change by enhancing helplessness and hopelessness (Pesa, Syre, T., & Jones, 2000; Strauss, 2000). Patients with emotional or behavioral disorders may need to see a psychologist or psychiatrist individually who can evaluate for and treat the issues (Vila et al., 2004). Psychologist-led group therapy sessions for the child and/or the caregivers can also be helpful in providing support and positive peer modeling for these children and their families (Eissa & Gunner, 2003). If significant family stress or negative family dynamics are present, a referral for family therapy may also be necessary.

The child's view on their treatment process is important. Significant predictors of weight loss were found to include the child's beliefs regarding personal control over weight, perceived difficulty of losing weight, attribution of obesity to their own medical problems or family problems, and perceived willingness of family members to diet (Uzark, Becker, Dielman, & Rocchini, 1987).

It is important to highlight the level of motivation as a critical component in treatment of overweight children. Individuals have varying degrees of motivation to change. The importance of motivation in enhancing the participation of obese children in exercise activities (McWhorter, Wallmann, & Alpert, 2003; Sallis et al., 2000) and in making healthier nutritional choices has been established (Carruth & Skinner, 2001). Studies show that being in the preparation/action stage of change suggests high motivation to make changes (Rhee et al., 2005). Multiple discussions with the patient and family often need to occur before a patient becomes ready to make changes. In addition, motivators for patients may be different. Patients can be motivated by increased athleticism, appearance, or social acceptance, which should be taken into account when having these discussions and deciding on goals.

Sociocultural Factors Affecting Treatment

Although rates of childhood obesity among the general population are alarmingly high, the rate is still higher in ethnic minority and low-income communities (Kumanyika & Greer, 2006). Obstacles cited as barriers to physical activity are unsafe streets, dilapidated parks, and lack of facilities. In Hispanic youths, barriers in the school system included lack of facilities, equipment, and trained staff for physical education (Thompson et al., 2001). Hispanic children are more sedentary than white children (Mirza et al., 2004) and resultantly overweight (Ritchie, Ivey, Woodward-Lopez, & Crawford, 2003).

Beyond the familial and personal factors, several sociocultural factors are known to impact nutritional and activity behaviors. Multiple studies have looked at and cited increased high-energy/low-cost foods including carbohydrates (Nicklas, Yang, Baranowski, Zakeri, & Berenson, 2003; Nielsen, Bjørnsbo, Tetens, & Heitmann, 2005), fats, and sugars (Nicklas et al., 2003; Troiano, Briefel, Carroll, & Bailostosky, 2000) as causes of childhood obesity. Many foods thought to be central to a healthy diet are perceived by some caregivers as too costly (Omar et al., 2001). The good taste, convenient preparation, and lower cost of foods with refined grains, added sugars, and added fats increase consumption of these foods (Drewnowski & Darmon, 2005; Drewnowski & Specter, 2004).

Some neighborhood environments have limited access to fruits and vegetables (Sallis & Glanz, 2006). Restaurants often provide large portion sizes, thus increasing intake of unhealthy foods and modeling unhealthy portion sizes for children (Young & Nestle, 2003). This is in comparison to nutrient-dense lean meats, fish, and fruits and vegetables, all of which cost more per serving and are further impacted by a lower satiation rate.

Lack of neighborhood safety may be a barrier to physical activity, causing significant anxiety in inner-city parents (Weir, Etelson, & Brand, 2006), and may be associated with an increased risk of overweight (Lumeng, 2005). One study involving 20 large U.S. cities showed mothers' perceptions of neighborhood safety to be related to their children's television-viewing time (Burdette & Whitaker, 2005). Screen time has been shown to have a positive relationship with an elevated BMI in children (Andersen et al., 1988; Proctor et al., 2003; Salmon, Campbell, & Crawford, 2006).

In addition, peers exert increasing influence on children and adolescents and ostracize those who are different. Young children are less willing to engage an obese peer in physical activities (Bell & Morgan, 2000), and overweight and obese children are more likely to be the victims of bullying as well as more likely to be the perpetrators of bullying behaviors than normal-weight peers (Janssen, Craig, Boyce, & Pickett, 2004). These peer reactions may lead to avoidance of physical activities that involve peers.

Goal Setting

Identifying and prioritizing goals play a central role in a weight loss program. Most frequently in children, a goal of weight maintenance is recommended by medical providers though there are medical situations that require a weight loss goal (see medical assessment section for details). For the majority of patients, however, a focus on actual weight is counterproductive. In fact, changes in specific eating and activity behaviors are more appropriate and realistic than weight management goals (Dietz, 1983) because changing the existing behaviors is more quickly identifiable, changes can be perceived more quickly than weight changes occur, and will likely have more immediate health benefits before weight loss occurs (Franz et al., 2002). Overweight children and their parents need reminding that even if they maintain their current weight, they will often grow in height, improving their BMI over time.

Once the primary emphasis on behavioral change is established, specific behavioral changes should be set as goals. For example, "decrease intake of drinks containing sugar such as juice, sweet tea, or soft drinks to 1 or less per week" or "move from 0 min of physical activity to 15 min per day." Initial goals should be few, focused, clearly defined, and devised so that they are achievable. This will build positive momentum toward further changes. Nutrition and activity behavioral change goals should be assessed regularly, and the goals refined and revised as needed over time.

Traditional behavioral modification techniques apply to nutrition and physical activity changes. Rewarding progress can increase compliance and motivation to maintain changes and set new goals. Starting slowly and shaping behaviors over time to reach an ultimate goal is another useful technique. Stimulus control techniques can also be helpful. Control techniques could include eating at the table and not in front of the TV or making sedentary activities such as time spent in front of a television or computer contingent upon completion of physical activity (Faith et al., 2001; Goldfield, Kalakanis, Ernst, & Epstein, 2000). This technique, called the *Premack Principle* (Premack, 1962) involves using a favorite, high-frequency activity as a reward for a behavior you would like to increase, such as physical activity. The patient is only allowed to engage in this favorite, high-frequency activity as a reward for achieving a daily goal.

Transcending the barriers to change involves lifestyle interventions. A multidisciplinary treatment approach is recommended: one that addresses family-centered treatment, nutrition and physical activity education, and behavior modification (Flodmark, Lissau, Moreno, Pietrobelli, & Widhalm, 2004). Coordination between the health-care professionals is important to avoid mixed messages given to patients and to learn what each discipline uniquely discovers about barriers. Combining perspectives and information should lead to a stronger treatment plan and greater treatment success.

It is critical to note that a positive approach toward patients and families throughout the assessment and treatment process is critical for success. Though working with individuals on their obesity can be challenging and frustrating if goals are not met and behavioral changes are not made, negative encounters with clinicians are rarely helpful but instead lead to patient/family discouragement, anger, and increased dropout rates. Instead, revising goals so that they are achievable for a particular family and shaping their progress slowly over time, with praise and positivity as they make each painstaking step, is more productive in the long run. Sometimes even deciding to wait until an individual or a family is ready to make changes is an acceptable way to maintain a positive rapport with a family in the face of low rates of goal achievement.

Conclusion

Health-care providers can learn the skills outlined here to help overweight and obese children and adolescents and their families achieve permanent, healthy lifestyle changes. It is a very rewarding work and can be incorporated as part of a busy general practice or as a specialty by itself. Using the medical, nutritional, physical activity, familial, psychological, and sociocultural assessments noted above, a comprehensive evaluation can be completed. This comprehensive assessment process will lead to (1) clearly definable goals and (2) the development of an individualized treatment plan that takes into account the unique combination of individual and family strengths as well as challenges, which is imperative in facilitating the achievement of success.

References

Adams, A., Quinn, R., & Prince, R. (2005). Low recognition of childhood overweight and disease risk among Native-American caregivers. *Obesity Research, 13*(1), 146–52.

American Academy of Pediatrics. (2003). Committee on nutrition, policy statement, prevention of pediatric overweight and obesity. *Pediatrics, 112*, 424–430.

American Dietetic Association. (2006). Position on the American Dietetic Association : Individual-, family-, school-, and community-based interventions for pediatric overweight. *Journal of the American Dietetic Association, 106*, June, 925–945.

Andersen, R.E., Crespo, C.J., Bartlett, S.J., Cheskin, L.J., & Pratt, M. (1988). Relationship of physical activity and television watching with body weight and level of fatness among children: Results from the third National Health and Nutrition Examinations Survey. *JAMA, 279*, 938–942.

Barlow, S.E., & Dietz, W.H., (1998). Obesity evaluation and treatment: Expert committee recommendations. *Pediatrics, 102*(3), e29.

Baughcum, A., Chamberlin, L., Deeks, C., Powers, S., & Whitaker, R. (2000). Maternal perceptions of overweight preschool children. *Pediatrics, 106*(6), 1380–6.

Bell, S., & Morgan, S. (2000). Children's attitudes and behavioral intentions toward a peer presented as obese: Does a medical explanation for the obesity make a difference? *Journal of Pediatric Psychology, 25*(3), 137–45.

Burdette, H., & Whitaker, R. (2005). A national study of neighborhood safety, outdoor play, television viewing, and obesity in preschool children. *Pediatrics, 116*(3), 657–62.

Calderon, K., Yucha, C., & Schaffer, S. (2005). Obesity-related cardiovascular risk factors: Intervention recommendations to decrease adolescent obesity. *Journal of Pediatric Nursing, 20*(1), 3–14.

Carruth, B., & Skinner, J. (2001). The role of dietary calcium and other nutrients in moderating body fat in preschool children. *International Journal of Obesity, 25*, 559–66.

Cason, K. (2006). Family mealtimes: More than just eating together. *Journal of American Dietetic Association, 106*(4), 532–3.

Cawley, J. (2006). Markets and childhood obesity policy. *Future of Children, 16*(1), 69–88.

Chen, J., & Kennedy, C. (2004). Family Functioning, Parenting Style, and Chinese Children's Weight Status. *Journal of Family Nursing, 10*(2), 262–79.

Dietz, W. (1983). Childhood obesity: Susceptibility, cause, and management. *Journal of Pediatrics, 103*, 676–86.

Dietz W.H., & Robinson T.H. (2005). Overweight children and adolescents. *NEJM, 352*(20), 2100–2109.

Drewnowski, A., & Darmon, N. (2005). The economics of obesity: Dietary energy density and energy cost. *American Journal of Clinical Nutrition, 82*(1), 265S–73.

Drewnowski, A., & Specter, S. (2004). Poverty and obesity: The role of energy density and energy costs. *American Journal of Clinical Nutrition, 79*(1), 6–16.

Eissa, M., & Gunner, K. (2003). Evaluation and management of obesity in children and adolescents. *Journal of Pediatrics Health Care, 18*, 35–8.

Epstein, L., Dearing, K., Handley, E., Roemmich, J., & Paluch, R. (2006). Relationship of mother and child food purchases as a function of price: A pilot study. *Appetite, 46*, 280–284.

Epstein, L., Paluch, R., Kalakanis, L., Goldfield, G., Cerny, F., & Roemmich, J. (2001). How much activity do youth get? A quantitative review of heart-rate measured activity. *Pediatrics, 108*(3), e44.

Epstein, L., Valoski, A., Wing, R., & McCurley, J. (1994). Ten-year outcomes of behavioral family-based treatment for childhood obesity. *Health Psychology, 13*(5), 373–83.

Epstein, L., Vito, D., & Anderson, K. (1996). Determinants of physical activity in obese children assessed by accelerometer and self-report. *Medical & Science in Sports & Exercise, 28*(9), 1157–64.

Expert Committee (2007). Assessment, Prevention and Treatment of Child and Adolescent Overweight and Obesity. http://www.amaassn.org/ama1/pub/upload/mm/433/ped_obesity_recs.pdf

Faith, M., Berman, N., Heo, M., Pietrobelli, A., Gallagher, D., Epstein, L., et al. (2001). Effects of contingent television on physical activity and television viewing in obese children. *Pediatrics, 107*(5), 1043–8.

Faulkner, M.S. (2002). Low income mothers of overweight children had personal and environmental challenges in preventing and managing obesity. *Evidence-Based Nursing, 5*, 27.

Flodmark, C.E., Lissau, I., Moreno, L., Pietrobelli, A., & Widhalm, K. (2004). New insights into the field of children and adolescents' obesity: The European perspective. *International Journal of Obesity, 28*(10), 1189–96.

Franz, M., Bantle, J., Beebe, C., Brunzell, J., Chiasson, J.L., Garg, A., et al. (2002). Evidence-based nutrition principles and recommendations for the treatment and prevention of diabetes and related complications. *Diabetes Care, 25*(1), 148–98.

Fulton, J.E., Garg, M., Galuska, D.A., Rattay, K.T., & Caspersen, C.J. (2004). Public health and clinical recommendations for physical activity and physical fitness: Special focus on overweight youth. *Sports Medicine, 34* (9), 581–599.

Gidding, S., Nehgme, R., Heise, C., Muscar, C., Linton, A., Hassink, S. (2004). Severe obesity associated with cardiovascular deconditioning, high prevalence of cardiovascular risk factors, diabetes mellitus/ hyperinsulinemia, and respiratory compromise. *Journal of Pediatrics, 144*, 766–9.

Golan, M., Weizman, A., & Fainaru, M. (1999). Impact of treatment for childhood obesity on parental risk factors for cardiovascular disease. *Preventive Medicine, 29*, 519–26.

Goldfield, G., Kalakanis, L., Ernst, M., & Epstein, L. (2000). Open-loop feedback to increase physical activity on obese children. *International Journal of Obesity, 24*(7), 888–92.

Jain, A., Sherman, S., Chamberlin, L., Carter, Y., Powers, S., & Whitaker, R. (2001). Why don't low-income mothers worry about their preschoolers being overweight? *Pediatrics, 107*(5), 1138–46.

Janssen, I., Craig, W., Boyce, W., & Pickett, W. (2004). Associations between overweight and obesity with bullying behaviors in school-aged children. *Pediatrics, 113*(5), 1187–94.

Jefferson, A. (2005). Breaking down barriers – examining health promoting behaviour in the family. Kellogg's Family Health Study 2005. *Nutrition Bulletin, 31*(1), 60–64.

Kumanyika, S., & Grier, S. (2006). Targeting interventions for ethnic minority and low-income populations. *Future Child, 16*(1), 187–207.

Levine, M., Ringham, R., Kalarchian, M., Wisniewski, L., & Marcus, M. (2001). Is family-based behavioral weight control appropriate for severe pediatric obesity? *International Journal of Eating Disorders, 30*(3), 318–28.

Lindsay, A., Sussner, K., Kim, J., & Gortmaker, S. (2006). The role of parents in preventing childhood obesity. *Future Child, 16*(1), 169–86.

Litwin, M., Sladowska, J., Antoniewicz, J., Niemirska, A., Wierzbicka, A., Daszkowska, J., et al. (2007). Metabolic abnormalities, insulin resistance, and metabolic syndrome in children with primary hypertension. *American Journal of Hypertension, 20*, 875–882.

Lumeng, J. (2005). What can we do to prevent childhood obesity? *Zero to Three, 25*(3), 13–9.

Marcus, D. (2004). Obesity and the impact of chronic pain. *Clinical Journal of Pain, 20*(3), 186–91.

McWhorter, J., Wallmann, H., & Alpert, P. (2003). The obese child: Motivation as a tool for exercise. *Journal of Pediatric Healthcare, 17*(1), 11–7.

Mirza, N., Kadow, K., Palmer, M., Solano, H., Rosche, C., & Yanovski, J. (2004). Prevalence of overweight among inner city Hispanic-American children and adolescents. *Obesity Research, 12*, 1298–310.

Must, A., & Strauss, R.S. (1999). Risks and consequences of childhood and adolescent obesity. *International Journal of Obesity & Related Metabolic Disorders, 23*(suppl 2), S2–S11.

National High Blood Pressure Education Program Working Group on High Blood Pressure in Children and Adolescents (2004). The Fourth report on the diagnosis, evaluation, and treatment of high blood pressure in children and adolescents. *Pediatrics, 114*, 555–576.

Nicklas, T., Yang, S., Baranowski, T., Zakeri, I., & Berenson, G. (2003). Eating patterns and obesity in children: The Bogalusa heart study. *American Journal of Preventive Medicine, 25*(1), 9–16.

Nielsen, B., Bjørnsbo, K., Tetens, I., & Heitmann, B. (2005). Dietary glycaemic index and glycaemic load in Danish children in relation to body fatness. *British Journal of Nutrition, 94*(6), 992–7.

Omar, M., Coleman, G., & Hoerr, S. (2001). Healthy eating for rural low-income toddlers: Caregivers' perceptions. *Journal of Community Health Nursing, 18*(2), 93–106.

Ogden, J., Reynolds, R., & Smith, A. (2006). Expanding the concept of parental control: A role for overt and covert control in children's snacking behaviour? *Appetite, 47*, 100–106.

Pesa, J., Syre, T., & Jones, E. (2000). Psychosocial differences associated with body weight among female adolescents: The importance of body image. *Journal of Adolescent Health, 26*(5), 330–7.

Pianosi, P.T., & Davis, H.S. (2004). Determinants of physical fitness in children with asthma. *Pediatrics, 113*(3), e225–e229.

Premack, D. (1962). Reversibility of the reinforcement relation. *Science, 136*, 255–7.

Proctor, M., Moore, L., Gao, D., Cupples, L., Bradlee, M., Hood, M., et al. (2003). Television viewing and change in body fat from preschool to early adolescence: The Framingham Children's Study. *International Journal of Obesity, 27*, 827–33.

Quattrin, T., Liu, E., Shaw, N., Shine, B., & Chiang, E. (2005). Obese children who are referred to the pediatric endocrinologist: Characteristics and outcome. *Pediatrics, 115*(2), 348–51.

Rhee, K., DeLago, C., Arscott-Mills, T., Mehta, S., & Davis, R. (2005). Factors associated with parental readiness to make changes for overweight children. *Pediatrics, 116*(1). e94–101.

Rhee, K., Lumeng, J., Appugliese, D., Kaciroti, N., & Bradley, R. (2006). Parenting styles and overweight status in first grade. *Pediatrics, 117*(6), 2047–54.

Ritchie, L., Ivey, S., Woodward-Lopez, G., & Crawford, P. (2003). Alarming trends in pediatric overweight in the United States. *Soz Praventivmed, 48*(3), 168–77.

Sallis, J., & Glanz, K. (2006). The role of built environments in physical activity, eating, and obesity in childhood. *Future Child, 16*(1), 89–108.

Sallis, J., Prochaska, J., & Taylor, W. (2000). A review of correlates of physical activity of children and adolescents. *Medicine & Science in Sports & Exercise, 32*(5), 963–75.

Salmon, J., Campbell, K., & Crawford, D. (2006). Television viewing habits associated with obesity risk factors: A survey of Melbourne schoolchildren. *Medical Journal of Australia, 184*(2), 64–7.

Schaub, B., & von Mutius, E. (2005). Obesity and asthma: What are the links? *Current Opinion Allery Clinical Immunology, 5* (2), 185–93.

Schwimmer, J.B., Deutsch, R., Rauch, J.B., Behling, C., Newbury, R., & Lavine, J.E. (2003). Obesity, insulin resistance, and other clinicopathological correlates of pediatric nonalcoholic fatty liver disease. *Journal of Pediatrics, 143*: 500–5.

Sothern, M., Hunter, S., Suskind, R., Brown, R., Udall, J., & Blecker, U. (1999). Motivating the obese child to move: The role of structured exercise in pediatric weight management. *South Medical Journal, 92*(6), 577–84.

Stefan, M., Hopman, W., & Smythe, J. (2005). Effect of activity restriction owing to heart disease on obesity. *Archives of Pediatric Adolescent Medicine, 159*(5), 477–81.

Strauss, R., & Knight, J. (1999). Influence of the home environment on the development of obesity in children. *Pediatrics, 103*(6), e85–92.

Strauss, R. (2000). Childhood obesity and self-esteem. Pediatrics, *105*(1), e15–9.

Strong, J.P., Malcom, G.T., Newman, W.P., & Oalmann, M.C. (1992). Early lesions of atherosclerosis in childhood and youth: National history and risk factors. *Journal of American College of Nutrition 11*(suppl), 51S–54S.

Tachdijian, M.O. (2002). *Pediatric orthopedics* (2nd edn., pp. 711–59) Philadelphia, PA: WB Saunders Co.

Thompson, J., Davis, S., Gittelsohn, J., Going, S., Becenti, A., Metcalfe, L., et al. (2001). Patterns of physical activity among American Indian children: An assessment of barriers and support. *Journal of Community Health: The Publication for Health Promotion and Disease Prevention, 26*(6), 407–21.

Treuth, M., Butte, N., Adolph, A., & Puyau, M. (2004). A longitudinal study of fitness and activity in girls predisposed to obesity. *Medicine & Science in Sports & Exercise, 36*(2), 198–204.

Troiano, R., Briefel, R., Carroll, M., & Bailostosky, K. (2000). Energy and fat intakes of children and adolescents in the United States: Data from the National Health and Nutrition Examination Surveys. *American Journal of Clinical Nutrition, 72*(Suppl), 1343S–53S.

Uzark, K., Becker, M., Dielman, T., & Rocchini, A. (1987). Psychosocial predictors of compliance with a weight control intervention for obese children and adolescents. *Journal of Compliance in Health Care, 2*(2), 167–78.

Vila, F., Zipper, E., Dabbas, M., Bertrand, C., Robert, J., Ricour, C., et al. (2004). Mental disorders in obese children and adolescents. *Psychosomatic Medicine, 66*(3), 387–94.

Vincer, R.M., Segal, T.Y., Lichtarowicz-Krynska, E., & Hindmarsh, P. (2005). Prevalence of the insulin resistance syndrome in obesity, *Archives of Disease in Childhood, 90*, 10–14.

Ward-Begnoche, W., & Gance-Cleveland, B. (2005). Promoting behavioral change in overweight youth. *Journal of Pediatric Health Care, 19*(5), 31–28.

Weir, L., Etelson, D., & Brand, D. (2006). Parents' perceptions of neighborhood safety and children's physical activity. *Preventive Medicine, 43*, 212–217.

Wrotniak, B., Epstein, L., Paluch, R., & Roemmich, J. (2004). Parent weight change as a predictor of child weight change in family-based behavioral obesity treatment. *Archives of Pediatric Adolescent Medicine, 158*(4), 342–7.

Young, K.L. (2005). Treating overweight children and adolescents in the clinic. *Clinical Pediatrics, 44* (8), 647–653.

Young, L., & Nestle, M. (2003). Expanding portion sizes in the US marketplace: Implications for nutrition counseling. *Journal of American Dietetic Association, 103*(2), 231–4.

Young-Hyman, D., Schlundt, D., Herman-Wenderoth, L., & Bozylinski, K. (2003). Obesity, appearance, and psychosocial adaptation on young African American children. *Journal of Pediatric Psychology, 28*(7), 463–72.

Young-Hyman, D., Schlundt, D.G., Herman, L., De Luca, F., & Counts, D. (2001). Evaluation of the insulin resistance syndrome in 5- to 10-year-old overweight/obese African-American children. *Diabetes Care, 24*, 1359–64.

Zametkin, A., Zoon, C., Klein, H., & Munson, S. (2004). Psychiatric aspects of child and adolescent obesity: A review of the past 10 years. *Journal of the American Academy of Child and Adolescent Psychiatry*, 43(2), 134–50.

Chapter 2
Practical Guidelines for Childhood Obesity Interventions

K. Beth Yano, Jenny Ebesutani, Christina Lu and Dariann Choy

About 25 million kids and teens in the United States are overweight or obese.

Unless we take action now to reverse this alarming trend, we're in danger of raising the first generation of American children who will live sicker and die younger than their parents' generation...

Robert Wood Johnson Foundation Newsletter, April 2007.

Childhood obesity is a growing global epidemic and a serious US public health threat impacting toddlers through teens in all 50 states across all socioeconomic and ethnic groups, though disproportionately affecting African American, Hispanic, American Indian, and Pacific Islander subgroups (Koplan, Liverman, & Kraak, 2005). Although there are genetic and biological factors related to childhood obesity, evidence indicates that modifiable environmental influences and learned behaviors significantly contribute to obesity and its rising rates (Jelalian & Mehlenbeck, 2003; Koplan et al., 2005). An increasing number of government, health, and private entities have responded to this crisis through efforts to fund and/or provide research and programs to address childhood obesity and related medical, psychological, social, and economic consequences (Huang & Horlick, 2007; Koplan et al., 2005). Thus it is an opportune time to present information and guidelines in support of the development of effective, efficient, and meaningful multi-level interventions to address childhood obesity.

Why Intervene with Children?

Over the past few decades, there has been a steady increase in the number of children who are overweight and at-risk for overweight (BMI at or above the 95th percentile for age and gender and 85th–94th percentile BMI, respectively). According to National Health and Nutrition Examination Survey (NHANES) results, the prevalence of overweight in children and adolescents ages 2- to 19-year-olds significantly increased from 13.9% in 1999 to 17.1% in 2004 (Ogden et al., 2006). Additionally, overweight status in childhood and adolescence is predictive of overweight and obesity in adulthood (Jelalian & Mehlenbeck, 2003) with estimates that about 75% of overweight adolescents will be overweight as adults

K.B. Yano (✉)
Child Psychology Service, Department of Psychology, Tripler Army Medical Center, Honolulu, HI, USA

L.C. James, J.C. Linton (eds.), *Handbook of Obesity Intervention for the Lifespan*,
DOI 10.1007/978-0-387-78305-5_3, © Springer Science + Business Media, LLC 2009

(Koplan et al., 2005). The physical, emotional, social, and healthcare costs associated with adult obesity are well documented (Flegal, Carroll, Ogden, & Johnson, 2002; Koplan et al., 2005; Sherwood & Jeffery, 2007) and efforts to intervene at younger ages can help to limit negative outcomes.

The need for prevention and intervention strategies is underscored by negative short-term and long-term medical, emotional, social, and economic consequences experienced by overweight children. Although many of the medical consequences of childhood obesity may not become evident until adulthood, there may be immediate medical sequelae affecting multiple organ systems among some youth, particularly those who are more severely overweight, and include glucose intolerance and insulin resistance, type II diabetes mellitus, hypertension, dyslipidemia, hepatic steatosis, cholelithiasis, sleep apnea, menstrual abnormalities, impaired balance, and orthopedic problems (Koplan et al., 2005). Psychosocial correlates of childhood obesity may include low self-esteem and depression among overweight school-aged children, particularly those who present for obesity treatment (Koplan et al., 2005). More consistent findings have been found regarding the presence of negative body image and physical appearance self-worth in school-aged children (Jelalian & Mehlenbeck, 2003). Decreased social competence and increased social problems, including difficulty with peer relations, teasing, discrimination, and social marginalization, are also related to obesity in childhood (Jelalian & Mehlenbeck, 2003). In addition, growing economic costs of childhood obesity have been identified, as estimates of obesity-related annual hospital costs for children and adolescents more than tripled during a recent 20-year period, increasing from $35 million in 1979–1981 to $127 million in 1997–1999 (Koplan et al., 2005). This dramatic increase in economic costs was related to the increasing percentage of hospital services for childhood obesity-related disease, including type II diabetes mellitus, gallbladder disease, and sleep apnea (Koplan et al., 2005).

Finally, prevention and early intervention strategies make good sense given the reported difficulties in maintaining weight loss in adulthood as well as the increasing body of literature supporting the short- and long-term efficacy of behavioral treatment for obesity in children, particularly between the ages of 8 and 12 (Epstein, 2003; Jelalian & Saelens, 1999). Fortunately, growing awareness of the need to effectively intervene with obesity among children is reflected in an increasing number of grants for childhood obesity research and interventions by both public and private organizations, such as the National Institute of Health (NIH), which funds 90% of obesity research in the United States (Huang & Horlick, 2007) and the Robert Wood Johnson Foundation, which has recently committed $500 million to address childhood obesity (Robert Wood Johnson Foundation, 2007).

What Factors Do We Need to Consider When Designing Child Obesity Interventions?

Childhood obesity is a complex problem, influenced by numerous factors and requiring multiple solutions across multiple systems. Genetic, biological, emotional, family, social, cultural, and environmental factors are recognized as contributors to childhood obesity (Jelalian & Mehlenbeck, 2003). More specifically, the alarming increase in childhood obesity appears to be connected to living in an obesogenic society with increasing social, cultural, and technological changes that lead to unhealthy lifestyles (Epstein, Paluch, Roemmich, & Beecher, 2007). Recognition and consideration of these social, environmental, and cultural factors impacting childhood obesity are critical to the development of effective child obesity interventions. Additionally, it is important to consider the child's and family's level of motivation to change as this factor can determine the success or failure of any given intervention.

Social–Ecological Model

Social–ecological models emphasize strong bi-directional influences between individuals and their environment to include family, school, cultural, community, and societal systems and the related importance of intervening at multiple levels to maximize change across systems (Bronfenbrenner, 1979; Kazak, 1989). This is particularly true for children who have limited control over these larger systems (Economos & Irish-Hauser, 2007). Additionally, preventive and public health approaches assert the need to intervene across all levels to effectively promote healthy lifestyle behaviors, support long-lasting behavior change, and shift social and cultural norms in favor of healthy lifestyles (Koplan et al., 2005).

Childhood obesity research indicates strong empirical support for behavioral-based interventions promoting healthy lifestyles (Bagby & Adams, 2007; Johnston & Steele, 2007) with the following conditions deemed important to maintaining healthy behaviors (Bagby & Adams, 2007; Epstein, Paluch, Kilanowski, & Raynor, 2004):

- available and accessible healthy foods;
- available and accessible options for moderate to vigorous physical activities;
- built-in environmental/structural support for lifestyle physical activity;
- ability to limit sedentary behaviors;
- healthy role models encouraging and modeling healthy eating and activity;
- positive encouragement and reinforcement of healthy behaviors.

Specific strategies to promote these conditions, across systems, are outlined in Table 2.1. These recommendations are culled from current child obesity research and practice literature (Ashe et al., 2007; Bagby & Adams, 2007; Economos & Irish-Hauser, 2007; Epstein et al., 2004; Peterson & Fox, 2007). Ideally, interventions would occur across all levels to address multiple needs. However, in reality, healthcare providers need to make informed choices about how to maximize positive change with specific factors and levels given our abilities, resources, funding, and population access.

Cultural Issues

Consideration of multi-cultural factors is essential in the development of childhood obesity interventions, given the increasing diversity of the US population, the influence of multi-cultural factors (i.e., ethnicity, socioeconomic status, geographical location, gender) on childhood obesity, as well as the recent changes in sociocultural norms regarding health-related behaviors due to societal changes in the pace of life, media/marketing practices, technological advances, and child safety concerns.

This section will provide a brief overview of cultural considerations that may inform childhood obesity interventions and is not intended to be an extensive review. Please refer to additional sources for more in-depth reviews of multi-cultural issues related to obesity interventions (Davis, Northington, & Kolar, 2000; Economos & Irish-Hauser, 2007;

Table 2.1. Social–ecological change strategies to support healthy lifestyle behaviors among children

Needs	Home–family	School	Neighborhood–community	Society
Available and accessible healthy foods	Keep healthy foods more visible, on counter Eliminate/limit unhealthy foods in home Eat more meals at home Choose restaurants with healthy food choices	Access to healthy, balanced school meals and snacks Eliminate soda and junk food from vending machines Add healthy choices (i.e., fruit, water) to vending machines Clean, accessible water fountains	Allow adequate zoning for agriculture activities Develop garden plots for neighborhoods with limited land space Support organization of local "farmers markets" Limit unhealthy "fast food" establishments	Require clear nutritional information for all foods Tax incentive for production and sales of healthy food choices Tax costs for production and sales of unhealthy foods
Available and accessible options for moderate to vigorous physical activities	Outdoor play area Accessible activity equipment Organized sports/athletic involvement Give activity-based gifts	Maintain adequate physical education (PE) time Include moderate to vigorous physical activities during PE time Allow adequate recess time throughout day Allow access to adequate playground equipment and other activity-based structures Distribute adequate number of balls, jump ropes, and other equipment for play Organize school sports teams	Sports and athletic leagues Safe and accessible public play areas —parks, fields, ball courts, gymnasiums, pools Encourage development of healthy activity-based child options (i.e., zoos, water parks, miniature golf courses, martial arts centers, dance groups)	Funding and/or tax incentives for development of activity-based child/family programs and establishments Media campaigns
Built-in environmental/structural support for lifestyle physical activity	Outdoor play, walks, and/or chores required daily Walk vs. drive when feasible	Adequate playground equipment and other activity-based structures Safe walking areas	Activity-friendly neighborhoods Safe parks, sidewalks and crosswalks Homes close to shops, community centers	Zoning regulations and financial incentives encouraging and reinforcing activity-based projects
Ability to limit sedentary behaviors	Limit TV and computer/video game playing to no more than 2 h/day and/or eliminate during weekdays	Include more activity-based instruction formats Create competition between students, classes or schools around the least recorded TV/electronic game times	Promotion of electronic-free playtime	Promotion of electronic-free playtime

Table 2.1. (continued)

Needs	Home–family	School	Neighborhood–community	Society
Healthy role models encouraging and modeling healthy eating and activity	Parents work toward improved eating and physical activity habits Parents host healthy birthday parties (balanced meal and physical activity)	Teachers and other school staff encourage and model healthy eating and physical activity behaviors Teachers encourage healthy foods at classroom/school festivities	Community-led healthy lifestyle programs (i.e., healthy food preparation, martial arts, sports, boys scouts/girl scouts)	Media campaigns Presentation of healthy behavior choices by popular public figures
Positive reinforcement of healthy behaviors	Praise for healthy behavior choices Individualized reward system	Develop recognition awards and incentives for healthy eating and activity behaviors for individuals, classes, and schools (i.e., class with the highest amount of recorded physical activity time earns a field trip School that earns greatest reduction in TV time contest earns extra playground equipment	Connect community privileges with participation in healthy lifestyle activities Organize community-based contests around health behaviors Recognize healthy behavior projects and accomplishments in local publications	Media support of healthy behaviors Money incentive for healthy behaviors (i.e., tax rebates, health insurance cost reductions)

Kumanyika, 2002, 2004) and of child obesity interventions with multi-cultural populations (Berry, Savoye, Melkus, & Grey, 2007; Chehab, Pfeffer, Vargas, Chen, & Irigoyen, 2007; Janicke et al., 2007; Sherwood & Jeffery, 2007).

Family ethnicity, worldviews, cultural values, and practices can impact many aspects of child obesity. Such values, beliefs, and practices often vary between different ethnic groups and may differ from Western norms. Modification of program objectives, content, and outcomes standards to address these cultural differences may promote engagement in treatment and long-term maintenance of behavior change among diverse families. Cultural adaptations to obesity interventions may include culturally relevant interactive and experiential learning activities, revision of written material to address language issues, and inclusion of cultural content regarding views of health, body image, dietary habits, physical activity, and coping strategies (Economos & Irish-Hauser, 2007; Kumanyika, 2002).

For example, family-based interventions, encouraging participation of parents, siblings and extended family members, are not only developmentally appropriate for children (given the strong influence of parents and other caregivers on behavior change among children) but also culturally appropriate for families holding collectivistic worldviews. Emphasizing family cohesion, collaborative goal setting, and teamwork may be particularly relevant for these families.

Also, it may be helpful to discuss cultural beliefs and practices regarding health and body image. Parents of certain ethnic minority groups (e.g., Black, Pacific Islanders) have shared that standards of beauty and health among their families differ from that of Western ideals of "thinness." Larger body size may be more accepted and/or expected among certain groups and may enhance social status (Kumanyika, 2004). The lack of stigma and acceptance of being overweight potentially influences family motivation to limit their children's weight. Such families may be motivated to engage in healthy behavior change for reasons other than the desire to achieve Western ideals of weight (e.g., physical health).

Thus, rather than focusing on the goal of weight loss, we encourage families to develop goals regarding specific lifestyle behaviors such as eating, physical activity, and coping skills (e.g., substitute water for sweet beverages, walk to park 5×/week). Such goals are more relevant, concrete, and understandable for children. These goals place less emphasis on culturally based standards of beauty and instead emphasize health. It is recommended that motivation for healthy lifestyle change focuses on the health benefits resulting from modest weight loss rather than holding Western norms as the ideal body image (Davis et al., 2000).

Similarly, sociopolitical and historical factors (i.e., Westernization) contributing to increasing prevalence of obesity should be acknowledged when working with indigenous populations who have experienced social, political, economic, and physical health loss/change as a result of increasing Westernization of the United States (Fitzpatrick-Nietschmann, 1983). Culture-based programs that incorporate indigenous beliefs, values, and practices have demonstrated some success with healthy behavior change (Economos & Irish-Hauser, 2007).

Beliefs and practices regarding food and nutrition also are strongly influenced by culturally mediated variables. Food and meals hold great social meaning for many families, particularly at family gatherings, and may be a central way of expressing love and care. Some families experience social expectations to eat large quantities of food as a sign of respect to individuals who have prepared and shared the food. Also, among families in low-income communities, caloric restriction may be associated with hunger and a sense of deprivation (Kumanyika, 2002). Interventions may include problem-solving discussions about ways to proactively avoid or respectfully respond to personal and social expectations regarding food. For example, families could make healthy modifications of ethnic foods, teach family members to cook healthily, and include these healthy food choices at family gatherings. It may be helpful to facilitate experiential cooking activities with families that include recipes and foods relevant to the families' ethnic groups with healthy modifications.

When working with diverse families, it is important to consider the degree of access to and comfort with community physical activity resources (Ashe et al., 2007). It is also important to consider cultural norms regarding acceptable physical activities for different ages and gender, such as children versus adults or women versus men (Kumanyika, 2004). There is some evidence of positive outcomes with child interventions utilizing culture-appealing physical activities (dance), particularly for girls (Sherwood & Jeffery, 2007).

Relatedly, there is additional evidence of differential treatment effects related to gender. Reviews of school-based interventions for childhood obesity (culture based and not) suggest differential treatment results for boys and girls with most interventions showing more favorable outcomes for girls (Cole, Waldrop, D'Auria, & Garner, 2006). In addition, a review of family-based child obesity treatments over the past 25 years indicates more favorable long-term outcomes for girls (Epstein et al., 2007).

Another cultural factor that may influence the success of obesity interventions is socio-economic status (SES; Kumanyika, 2004). Families with limited economic resources may have additional poverty-related stressors and less money, time, and coping resources to allow for modeling of and engagement in healthy eating and regular physical activity regimens (Kitzmann & Beech, 2006). These families may benefit from connection to additional resources and creative solutions to meet their basic needs and enhance ability to engage in healthy lifestyle behaviors. It also is important to acknowledge the prioritization of more "pressing" issues (e.g., finances, basic resources), rather than blaming or pathologizing families as having made poor choices or effort.

Geographic location also impacts the feasibility of successful behavior change. Communities vary in terms of availability of resources and environmental factors to support healthy lifestyle behavior change (Economos & Irish-Hauser, 2007). For example, rural communities tend to have higher poverty rates and limited access to important health-related resources—such as medical services; organized community sports, gyms, and safe parks; or stores with fresh and affordable produce and other healthy food choices (Janicke et al., 2007). Families living in these areas may require community-based programs that provide outreach and additional support to gain access to resources (e.g., afterschool programs, local organizations that promote physical activity for children) and creative alternatives to increase healthy lifestyle behaviors among families (Kumanyika, 2002).

In order to develop and implement cultural adaptations or culture-based programs for childhood obesity, it is essential for program facilitators to be aware of their own worldviews, cultural beliefs/values, and potential biases regarding lifestyle behaviors and obesity. Inclusion of multi-cultural staff and/or community leaders in the development and implementation of interventions may support recruitment efforts and initial "buy in" of diverse families (Ahina, 2003). In addition, though there may be differences in cultural beliefs, values, and behaviors between groups, it is also important to recognize within-group variability and explore the unique needs, goals, and resources of each family and family member.

Recent societal changes across the United States have contributed to increases in high-fat food consumption and sedentary lifestyles. For example, the faster pace of life and increase in single parent families have contributed to reductions in home-prepared meals and an increase in eating out and fast food consumption (Koplan et al., 2005). A National Institute of Health review concluded that these behaviors are risk factors for overweight in children (Peterson & Fox, 2007). Also, targeted media and marketing of high-fat foods for children has led to increased pressures to purchase these unhealthy foods (Koplan et al., 2005). Additionally technological advances involving computers, video games, and television options have contributed to an increasingly sedentary lifestyle. To counter the impact of these societal trends, interventions are needed to decrease fatty and fast food consumption, decrease portion sizes, decrease "screen time," and increase and/or introduce children to new physical behaviors and community-organized physical activities.

In addition, there is growing parental concern about child safety issues related to increasing size of communities and child predator threats. Some parents have become increasingly protective of their children, not allowing them to play outside and/or limiting community activities. In these cases, discussion with parents about fears, safety, and feasible solutions for physical activities is warranted.

The current US military involvement in the Middle East has contributed to increased stress as well as decreased resources (e.g., time, coping strategies) to attend to healthy lifestyle behaviors in some military families. Increased stressors paired with additional caregiving/household responsibilities often interfere with the family's ability to attend treatment and to implement healthy lifestyle behaviors. Thus, it has been helpful to include childcare or sibling treatment components as well as coping and stress management skills training in interventions for military families.

Ongoing research is needed to explore the impact of cultural/societal change on family health behaviors and to support interventions to counter the effects of our obesogenic society (Epstein et al., 2007; Peterson & Fox, 2007). In addition, research is needed to support the development of effective culturally mindful interventions given increasing prevalence of overweight and obesity among certain ethnic minority groups in the United States, such as Black, Latino, Native American, and Pacific Islander populations (Kumanyika, 2004; US Department of Health and Human Services, 2001), and research findings suggesting decreased efficacy of weight-loss interventions for ethnic minority populations versus Caucasian groups (Germann et al., 2007).

Stages of Change Model

Initiating and maintaining healthy behavior change can be a challenging process for families, particularly amidst the multitude of barriers to healthful lifestyles. Thus, it is essential to explore families' degree of readiness to change and intervene accordingly, rather than assume that all families presenting for treatment are immediately ready to engage in behavior change (Golan, 2006).

Prochaska and DiClemente (1983) developed the stages of change (or transtheoretical) model integrating key concepts from various theories to help describe and explain how individuals modify problem behaviors and/or acquire positive behaviors. They have identified six stages of change and 10 related processes of change. It is assumed that individuals vary in their readiness to change and may not always benefit from traditional action-oriented interventions. Research supports the multiple benefits of matching interventions with an individual's readiness to change status. Prochaska and Velicer (1997) posited, "Applied research has demonstrated dramatic improvements in recruitment, retention, and progress using stage-matched interventions and proactive recruitment procedures" (p. 38).

Precontemplation is described as the stage in which the individual is not intending to make any changes within the foreseeable future (6 months). They may be unaware about the consequences of their behaviors or they may have experienced failed attempts to change in the past. Contemplation is the stage in which there is intention to change within the next 6 months as individuals recognize a problem behavior and are aware of positive and negative consequences. There are often feelings of ambivalence about change and commitment which often lead to remaining stuck in this stage for long periods of time. In the preparation stage, individuals intend to change within the next month and often report making a few changes. The action stage involves individuals displaying specific, overt behavior change for at least 6 months. During the maintenance stage health behavior is consistent and individuals continue to work on sustained change and relapse prevention. Termination indicates successful maintenance of health behavior and confidence in ability to fully maintain behavior change, with the acknowledgment that an individual may experience relapse and return to previous stages with this non-linear model and therefore again require interventions.

Prochaska and DiClemente (1983) also identified 10 processes that facilitate change or movement from one stage to the next. A summary of these change processes are presented based on the writings of Prochaska and Velicer (1997). During the precontemplation stage, *consciousness raising* and *environmental reevaluation* processes may facilitate change by increasing awareness of the nature, causes, consequences, and reinforcers of the problem behavior (via public media campaigns, mailings, books, psychoeducational presentations and through consultation with medical providers, family, and friends) and by increasing awareness of how people impact their social and physical environments. For example, families in the precontemplation stage may benefit from learning about the consequences of childhood obesity and the impact of their home environment and family eating and activity patterns on child health behaviors. *Helping relationships* are a process of change that may be beneficial throughout all stages. A helping relationship provides an empathic, caring, trusting, and accepting environment that supports enhanced motivation. As providers, it is important to build rapport and strong therapeutic alliances to maximize the helping relationship role. It is also helpful for individuals to have a healthy support network of family, friends, and community resources.

Emotional arousal is one of the processes of change that can help individuals move out of precontemplation and contemplation stages to preparation and action stages. Experiencing a dramatic event such as watching an intense movie, role playing, and imaginative activities often elicits motivating emotions such as fear, worry, and guilt. *Self-reevaluation* can facilitate movement out of contemplation and involves cognitive and emotional evaluation of one's self-image and problem behavior. The aim is to help individuals counter ambivalence through realizing that their values are in conflict with their problematic behaviors. Techniques of self-reevaluation include clarifying essential values, using imagery, and interacting with healthy role models. In the preparation stage, individuals decide to make a commitment to change. The change process of *commitment* or *self-liberation* includes a willingness to act as well as the belief in one's ability to make changes. Many individuals experience anxiety as change can be challenging and threatening, and often benefit from anxiety-reducing strategies such as taking small steps, setting a date to take action, making the commitment known to family, friends, neighbors, and colleagues, and creating an individualized plan of action. *Social liberation* processes lead to increased healthy alternatives for individuals through enhanced community and societal support for behavior change. For example, salad bars in schools offer children alternatives that support healthier eating.

In the action stage, it is helpful to engage in the following processes of change: *countering, stimulus control*, and *contingency management. Countering* occurs when individuals substitute healthier behaviors for problem behaviors. For example, instead of watching television where there is a greater chance of snacking and being sedentary, children could ride a bicycle outside. *Stimulus control* involves restructuring the environment to decrease the likelihood of engaging in the problem behavior and increase the likelihood of engaging in healthy behaviors. For example, removing cues for unhealthy behaviors (e.g., removing snacks from view) and adding prompts or reminders for healthier alternatives (e.g., having easy access to physical game equipment) promote healthy behavior choices. *Contingency management* helps to shape healthy behaviors through the use of reinforcers.

It is important to note that the stage change theory is a non-linear model and individuals may move forward or backwards through stages over time. Also, individuals tend to make several attempts to change behaviors before being able to successfully manage and maintain behavior change over an extended period of time. A summary of change stages, change processes, and matched strategies for child obesity intervention is presented in Table 2.2, adapted from Prochaska and Velicer (1997).

Table 2.2. Matching stage of change status with appropriate strategies for child obesity

Stage of change	Process of change	Strategies for child obesity
Pre-contemplation	Consciousness raising	Media, books, informational handouts, psycho-educational workshops; Consultation with pediatricians and other healthcare providers
	Environmental reevaluation	Observe and review impact of environment on child's health behaviors
	Helping relationships	Support from family, peers, teachers, and providers
	Emotional arousal	Dramatic and documentary film media (e.g., Supersize Me); imagining their future health if they do not change; review of negative health consequences in their personal lives/families
Contemplation	Self-reevaluation	Clarify values, review self-image with and without desired behavior(s); evaluate pros and cons of behavior choices
Preparation	Commitment or self liberation	Create specific steps or plans of action; set a realistic date to start making changes, announce to family and friends plans to change
	Social liberation	Healthier alternatives (i.e., salad) for school lunches; expanded physical activity options—increase in PE requirements; additional recreational equipment at school and community parks
Action	Countering	Replace watching TV with engaging in an enjoyable physical activity; relaxation techniques to cope with stress and anxiety
	Stimulus control	Sweets and snacks removed from view; fruit on display in kitchen; weights strategically placed in home: TV locked
	Contingency management	Behavioral contracting (e.g., earning rewards for engaging in specific healthy behaviors); teach positive self-statements (e.g., "I'm doing a great job at eating a vegetable with dinner"); parents praising child for engaging in specific healthy behaviors
Maintenance		Continue to use above interventions and "booster sessions" to reinforce behavior change

What Can We Do? Practical Guidelines for Clinicians

The following practical guidelines are designed to inform and promote the development of creative, thoughtful, and effective clinical interventions. The guidelines are based on a review of the child obesity literature as well as child obesity treatment experiences at the Lean Family programs adapted from the Adult Lean (James, Folen, Page, Noce, & Britton, 1999; James et al., 1997) and Kids Lite Programs (Ahina, 2003) at Tripler Army Medical Center. Case illustrations are provided throughout to highlight practical application of these guidelines.

1. Assess needs of your target population and collaborate with complementary organizations, departments, and other resources in the development and implementation of appropriate interventions. The Lean Family programs at Tripler Army Medical Center (TAMC) were designed to meet the growing number of child referrals for obesity treatment—most of whom appeared to require additional information, support with the application of information, and modeling of effective goal setting, monitoring, and reinforcement of positive behavior change. Many referrals were seeking services different from traditional individual counseling as they had reached maximum benefit from this type of service. Thus the group-oriented Lean Family programs were developed to fulfill these unmet service needs. Partnering with other groups can enhance program scope and quality, maximize resources, prevent service overlaps, increase maintenance supports, and reduce funding for individual groups (due to pooled resources). At the Lean Family programs, we were able to partner with nutritional specialists who assisted with the development and presentation of nutritional information, the meal planning for camp meals, and funding for healthy food samples. It was a win–win situation as nutritionists were able to assist in powerful change-producing group formats, and other providers were able to learn from their expertise.

2. Develop referral, screening, and intake processes that will support the selection of participants who would likely benefit from planned intervention. Inform referral sources of the nature and scope of your interventions. Screen for medical and psychiatric conditions that may be primary causes of obesity or that may interfere with treatment and need to be addressed first or simultaneously (i.e., hypothyroidism, type II diabetes, major depression, anxiety disorders). Incorporate an informative "orientation session" during intake to increase families' understanding of program goals and expectations, and enhance providers' understanding of child/family goals and expectations. This process may serve to identify families whose goals/needs fit with the proposed program and lead to decreased attrition and increased satisfaction with the program (Germann, Kirschenbaum, & Rich, 2006).

   In the Lean Family programs, candidates routinely require medical review to screen for biological bases for obesity and to assess for the safety of mild to vigorous physical activity. The intake also includes measures to screen for psychological issues. A positive screen will lead to further exploration and action plans, as appropriate, ranging from concurrent active monitoring, individualized family support, or acceptance to the program after adequate treatment. Individualized support for families with these additional psychological needs has led to positive results including increased attendance, success with reaching behavioral goals, and reported satisfaction with program.

   The program has utilized a variety of orientation formats including over-the-phone program reviews, individual family sessions, and multi-family group presentations. Thus far, group orientation sessions allowing for exposure to and connection with other families have produced the best results in terms of improved attendance and family engagement in change processes. In addition, group orientations are more efficient and offer opportunities for staff to observe and prepare for intra-family dynamics that may impact behavior change.

3. Assess child and family readiness to change and select interventions that are appropriate and meaningful for their particular stages of change. Clinical interventions can be tailored to address various change stages. For example, one time psycho-educational presentations and workshops are suited to those in precontemplation and contemplation stages. It serves the purpose of "raising consciousness" and reviewing personal "pros and cons" of change for participants and spares providers an over-investment of resources. Those in preparation and action phases have momentum to change and are more likely to benefit from and be motivated to attend more frequent sessions (Prochaska & Velicer, 1997). A popular and effective arrangement includes an initial group orientation session followed by weekly group meetings that fade-out over time as participants advance through the change process. The typical structure for this type of program is 8–15 sessions within a 6–8-month period (Young, Northern, Lister, Drummond, & O'Brien, 2007). Those in the maintenance stage could benefit from intermittent monitoring checks and "booster sessions", as needed, to reinforce gains.

4. Utilize motivational interviewing techniques to support child/parent clarification of and movement through change stages. Change processes and related movement through stages are impacted by an individual's level of motivation. Practitioners can use motivational interviewing to help children and families process and work through their ambivalence about behavior change as well as challenges that they may face in later stages. The four principles of motivational interviewing (MI) include expressing empathy, developing discrepancy, rolling with resistance, and supporting self-efficacy (Miller & Rollnick, 2002). The practitioner creates a non-judgmental, accepting, and empathic environment in which individuals can openly express the positive and negative aspects about their behaviors. The role of the practitioner is not to offer advice or try to convince individuals to change. Rather, it involves supporting individuals in developing their own reasons for and against change and in understanding how their current behaviors affect their abilities to achieve their goals in life and maintain their core values. While practitioners generally limit questions and focus on reflecting, when working with children it may be necessary to ask more questions to elicit responses (Resnicow, Davis, & Rollnick, 2006). Although there is limited research on the use of motivational interviewing with childhood obesity, evidence for other health concerns have shown promising results. Furthermore, parents report being satisfied with motivational interviewing strategies utilized by pediatricians and registered dieticians (Resnicow et al., 2006).

5. Structure program to maximize attendance and benefit families. It is important to be mindful of families' abilities and limitations regarding attendance and participation in obesity interventions. Attendance is enhanced when programs take into account common logistical issues, such as geographical proximity of program, transportation, childcare for siblings, school schedules, and winter and summer breaks. Program adaptation to these variables may help to reduce family barriers to attendance, enhance program value, and increase active participation. For example, after learning that parents experienced difficulties with parent-group participation due to childcare responsibilities, we developed a concurrent sibling group designed to teach and promote healthy behaviors among family members. In addition, parking availability at our hospital has worsened over the years and families complained of circling upwards of 30 minutes to find a parking space; thus, we altered our schedule and location so that we met first for

physical activity exposure at the gym, which had ample parking, and then walked to the nearby hospital building for the remainder of group. These strategies increased attendance and retention of participants.

6. Utilize a family-based approach. Sustained behavior change in children requires the support and involvement of family. Multi-program reviews and long-term clinical research studies have indicated the efficacy of including families in the treatment of child obesity. Inclusion of family—particularly parents—in the change process enhances child behavior change and treatment outcomes (Epstein, 2003; Epstein et al., 2007; Jelalian & Mehlenbeck, 2003; Young et al., 2007). In fact, some studies have demonstrated efficacy of parent-only interventions (Golan, 2006; Kitzmann & Beech, 2006), highlighting the power of teaching parents to be the change agents for their children. The Lean Family program recognizes the importance and value of incorporating families in all aspects of child interventions, from intake through termination. Our goal is to provide families with the information and tools they will need to continue to guide and support healthy lifestyles for their children.

7. Utilize group formats. Comprehensive family-based behavioral treatment programs, consisting of group formats with an individualized focus for each family, have become primary forms of treatment for childhood obesity (Epstein et al., 2007). Various types of group formats are available, including multi-family groups, group treatment for children, and group treatment for parents and other primary caregivers. Group-only treatment for parents and children has been shown to be a particularly cost-effective approach with equal efficacy to a mixed approach involving both group and individual treatment. The group approach was found to be more cost-effective than the mixed approach in terms of decrease in percent overweight per dollar spent on treatment (Goldfield, Epstein, Kilanowski, Paluch, & Kogut-Bossler, 2001).

The advantages of group approaches include efficiency, cost-effectiveness, accountability, support, and group participation in more creative problem solving. The ongoing presence, support, and monitoring by other group members may provide each group member with a sense of accountability and motivation to continue attending treatment and engaging in healthy behavior change. The group format also allows for the sharing of multiple perspectives and concrete solutions to obstacles to behavior change. Suggestions from other group members may be particularly effective and influential, as they may hold a special type of credibility as compared with suggestions from group facilitators.

Additionally, the group format may provide children with a safe and enjoyable environment that promotes a greater sense of connection, engagement, and commitment. Children in earlier stages of change (i.e., precontemplation, contemplation) may benefit from the modeling and positive examples of other children who are engaging in active behavior change. In addition, children in active stages of change may benefit from serving as models and "helpers" for children in earlier stages of change. We have also found it helpful to include siblings in these child groups to support the generalization of healthy lifestyle behaviors in the home.

Parental involvement is an effective component of behavioral treatment for childhood obesity (Jelalian & Mehlenbeck, 2003). Parent groups can provide parents with information, group discussion, and group support with coping skills, problem-solving strategies, parenting skills, and behavior change strategies that promote healthy lifestyle behaviors in their children, their families, and themselves. Within the Lean Family program, parents have consistently reported satisfaction with the parent-group component, particularly the group discussions focused on emotional and psychological factors contributing to their children's lifestyle behaviors (i.e., "emotional eating") and discussion regarding problem-solving strategies to promote healthy behavior change.

When utilizing a group format, it is also essential to maintain an individualized focus on each family's unique goals, needs, and strengths. This may be done through individual family check-ins within or outside of group sessions. In the Lean Family program, we had the benefit of multiple facilitators that could provide individualized family support within multi-family group meetings. For example, following group presentation and discussion regarding behavioral goal setting and reinforcement, a "break-out" session is conducted where each family is paired with a facilitator to assist with refinement of behavior goals and reinforcement strategies.

8. A comprehensive curriculum can include information and applied practice with nutrition and healthy eating behaviors, physical activity, behavioral change strategies, emotional issues, coping and problem-solving skills, and stages of change and relapse prevention strategies.

   a. Nutrition and healthy eating behaviors. The Lean Family program introduces the importance of knowing *W*hen to eat, *H*ow to eat, the *A*mount to eat, and *T*ype of foods to eat (WHAT). Parents and children learn about nutritional requirements via the Food Guide Pyramid (US Department of Agriculture, 2005). They learn the value of eating smaller and more frequent balanced meals, eating at home, eating in a designated area without other activities, using smaller plates, chewing slowly, and drinking more water and less sugar-sweetened drink. Parents share ideas regarding economic and efficient ways to plan, shop, and prepare healthier meals. Both parents and children are exposed to a variety of healthy food alternatives through tasting of healthy ready-made snacks (e.g., low calorie chips/cookies, soy milk, indigenous fruits) and prepared foods (e.g., whole wheat vegetarian spaghetti, tofu pie). The efficacy of these strategies is reported in a variety of studies (Howard, 2007; Jelalian & Mehlenbeck, 2003; Peterson & Fox, 2007).

   b. Physical activity. Reducing sedentary behaviors and increasing physical activity have been related to improved health outcomes and reduction in risk for childhood obesity (Jelalian & Mehlenbeck, 2003; Peterson and Fox, 2007). Reduction of sedentary behaviors tends to promote more positive outcomes by decreasing unhealthy eating behaviors paired with sedentary behaviors and by increasing time to engage in active behaviors (Epstein et al., 2004). The Lean Family program introduces families to the benefits of stretching, aerobic, and anaerobic exercises and incorporates experiential exposure to a variety of physical activities including walking, jogging, swimming, jump rope, weight lifting, and competitive games. Families discuss typical barriers to physical activity, including time constraints, preference for sedentary behavior (television, internet, and video games), lack of involvement in organized sports, and embarrassment about participation in competitive sports or physical activity. Families also share helpful suggestions to address these barriers to include (1) have a specific plan to increase physical activity; (2) plan activities the whole family can participate in; (3) limit television, computer, and video game time; (4) incorporate minor changes in daily activities, such as walking instead of driving, parking farther from the designation, taking the stairs instead of the elevator; (5) explore additional community-based activities; (6) plan parties and vacations around movement and play; and (7) buy birthday/holiday gifts that promote activity.

   c. Behavioral change strategies to include self-monitoring, stimulus control, goal setting, behavioral contracting, shaping, positive reinforcement, and modeling.

Behavioral theory assumes that behaviors are learned and that learning occurs through classical conditioning, operant conditioning, and/or social learning (Bandura, 1986). Maladaptive behavior can be unlearned and more adaptive behavior can be learned. In treating obesity, the goal is to systematically change eating patterns, physical activity, and other behaviors that maintain obesity (Drohan, 2002). Thus it is beneficial to teach the following behavioral concepts and strategies to promote behavior change (Cole et al., 2006).

1. *Self-monitoring.* In order to modify dietary, physical activity, and emotional coping habits, children's existing behavior patterns need to be identified. Self-monitoring may help increase awareness of specific behaviors as well as identify a child's particular strengths and weakness (Evans & Sullivan, 1993). Evidence also suggests that consistent child self-monitoring leads to improved weight loss outcomes and that self-monitoring by parents increases self-monitoring by children (Germann et al., 2007). While monitoring helps to assess problem behaviors and tailor interventions, it can also serve to track progress and goal attainment. Often times, simply engaging in self-monitoring leads to positive changes. Children can record daily food and drink intake, physical activity, and mood ratings. Depending on the child's developmental level, it may be necessary to rely on parents to complete daily logs for more accurate reports. At the same time, it is important to involve children in the process and create opportunities that allow them to utilize their abilities. For example, children may be able to draw what they ate each day or may be able to carry a camera to take pictures of each meal before they eat. Monitoring may be more feasible if done for specific time periods or alternately, one weekday and one weekend, rather than daily.

2. *Stimulus control.* There is often a relationship between eating and the environment or situation in which eating occurs (Drohan, 2002; Economos & Irish-Hauser, 2007). Therefore, it is important to help families identify environmental triggers of unhealthy eating habits and alter environments to promote healthy eating. Some suggested alterations include shopping from a grocery list and avoiding strategically placed high-fat/high-sugar foods, limiting purchase of unhealthy food and drink, placing healthy foods on accessible countertops, limiting eating to one room, and keeping meal food on the countertop rather than within reach at the meal table (Golan, 2006). Similarly, stimulus control can lead to reductions in sedentary behaviors and increases in physical activity (Bagby & Adams, 2007; Epstein et al., 2004). For example, parents can limit sedentary behaviors by placing time limits on television and computer use and/or removing these machines from bedrooms. In addition, physical activities can be embedded in family routines, and prompts for physical activity (e.g., sports equipment) can be placed around the home environment.

3. *Goal setting/shaping/behavioral contracting.* Goal setting is a very important process that can set the stage for significant positive changes or, alternatively, lead to disappointment and discontinuation. Within the Lean Family programs, families learn about goal-setting processes and are supported in the development of behavior change plans with specific goals for eating, physical activity, and coping behaviors. Children are fully involved in the planning process. Goals are specific, measurable, and attainable. Families are encouraged to start small, build in success, and increase expectations as one progresses (shaping). An agreement or behavioral contract is recommended to clarify goals, establish rewards, and increase "buy-in" (Drohan, 2002).

4. *Positive reinforcement.* Reinforcements for engaging in healthy behaviors and for *not* engaging in unhealthy behaviors can lead to increased weight loss percentages (Epstein et al., 2004; Jelalian & Mehlenbeck, 2003). In the Lean Family programs, appropriate reinforcement strategies are taught to parents and incorporated in intervention processes.

5. *Modeling.* Children tend to model, or imitate, the behaviors of those around them. Parents, siblings, peers, and other significant persons have an influence on what children choose to eat or what types of activities they engage in (Drohan, 2002). Thus it is critical to teach parents the value of demonstrating healthy lifestyle behaviors including healthy eating, regular physical activity, and appropriate coping with emotions and stress. In addition, it is beneficial to expose children to new foods and activities on a regular basis thereby increasing healthy options and preferences.

d. Emotional issues. There is growing evidence supporting the link between obesity, perceived stress, and emotional eating in youth (Nguyen-Rodriguez, Chou, Unger, & Spruijt-Metz, 2008). In addition, depression, low self-esteem, negative body image, and self-worth are associated with childhood obesity (Jelalian & Mehlenbeck, 2003; Koplan et al., 2005). Therefore the Lean Family program incorporates modules to illuminate emotional-based eating and to offer emotional-cognitive support strategies to families. Families have consistently provided positive feedback regarding these modules, reporting that they have found them helpful in understanding and addressing their child's emotional and stress-related issues.

e. Healthy coping and problem-solving skills. Although there is limited research regarding the efficacy of coping and problem-solving skills with childhood obesity treatments, a recent study (Berry et al., 2007) with multi-ethnic families supported the use of coping skills training (CST) which included communication, cognitive behavioral techniques, and social problem-solving skills. When provided to obese parents, CST led to enhanced outcomes in an established program for overweight multi-ethnic youth (Berry et al., 2007). In addition, family-based child obesity treatment research suggests the value of exploring the use of parent coping skills to enhance child obesity outcomes (Golan, 2006; Kitzmann & Beech, 2006).

f. Stages of change and relapse prevention strategies. The Lean Family programs have adopted the strategy of teaching families about stages of change and related processes. As a result, families appear better able to identify and successfully work through stages. Families learn to identify barriers to maintaining behavior change, prepare for triggers, and plan for falls (Ahina, 2003). Empirical research regarding the effectiveness of these techniques is needed.

9. Utilize behavior change strategies in the intervention process. Using behavior change techniques in the intervention process serves to reinforce general learning as well as model the very strategies that we teach families. For example, in the Lean Family programs, *self-monitoring* is promoted through regular reviews of individual child behavior logs. *Goal setting* and *contracting* are modeled through individualized support for the development and implementation of behavior plans and contracts. In addition, *positive reinforcement* is modeled through a program token system offering rewards for program attendance, completion of behavior logs, and success with behavior goals. Finally, healthy eating, physical activity, and coping strategies are modeled through experiential modules.

10. Utilize multi-modal teaching with emphasis on experiential-based activities and consideration of the developmental levels of participants. Presenting information and activities in multiple modalities—visual, verbal, and kinesthetic—addresses the needs of children (and adults) with differing learning styles and supports repetitive learning that enhances retention. Kinesthetic, experiential-based learning is a particularly effective teaching approach because such "hands-on-learning" helps to make constructs concrete, understandable, and meaningful for children, thereby enhancing their learning and behavior change processes. These experiential learning approaches also allow for modification according to children's developmental and cognitive levels of functioning. School-aged children may be better able to learn through exploration with concrete interactive activities because they have not yet developed the abstract reasoning abilities and verbal skills that are needed to process experiences through abstract thought (Piaget, 1962). Action-oriented methods of learning incorporate imagery, action, and direct interpersonal experience with the problem situation, exposing children to concrete and tangible aspects of a problem behavior, habit, or thought. These experiential approaches help to produce insight through action (Blatner, 2001). This experiential learning process also increases the meaningfulness and applicability of learned skills and behaviors, thereby promoting the generalization of new skills to children's daily life experiences.

    Experiential activities within-group settings provide further benefits to children including opportunities to clarify their own thoughts, feelings, and challenges; become aware of shared struggles; and collectively discover creative solutions. In addition, these interactive activities promote strong group cohesion and identification of additional sources of support among the young group members.

    Examples of multi-modal experiential teaching of nutrition within the Lean Family programs include

    a. Nutrition and meal-planning: activities such as verbal presentation of the food pyramid; visual viewing of portion sizes and types of food for each food category; mixed parent–child teams draw well-balanced meals on paper plates with color crayons and then share their rationale for healthy meal choices to the group;
    b. Increasing awareness of "Empty Calorie" drinks: verbal discussion of the negative consequences of excess sugar and needless sugar/calories that are hidden in common child drinks; and identifying the amount of sugar in various beverages by measuring the number of teaspoons of sugar into plastic cups;
    c. Simple exposure to new foods: discussion of healthy alternative food choices; presentations of healthy food alternative for children and adults to taste; and demonstration and participation with cooking healthy food alternatives.

    Parents and children reported that they have enjoyed and benefited from these informative and interactive experiences.

11. Incorporate and encourage the use of community resources to increase exposure to varied healthy lifestyle choices related to physical activity, eating, stress management, and coping strategies. Actual exposure to and practice with these healthy behaviors in community settings can support interest in, accessibility to, and maintenance of healthy lifestyle choices. Ideas include exposure to

    a. Physical activity: simple hikes; a walk in the park; playing basketball, volleyball, frisbee, jump rope, or hopscotch; visits to the zoo, aquarium, ice-skating rink, and fitness gyms;

b. Healthy foods and locations to obtain them: visits to community gardens, farmers' markets, healthy food stores, or general restaurants with healthy food choices;
c. Stress management and healthy coping skills: walk at the park, beach, or mall; watching a funny movie; martial arts classes; art classes; visit to art museum; yoga in the park.

12. Collect quantitative and qualitative outcome data (i.e., pre-post measures, satisfaction and feedback surveys) to evaluate the program and critically inform the development of future interventions. Childhood obesity programs have generally targeted changes in weight or BMI status via interventions promoting dietary changes, increased physical activity, and decreased sedentary behaviors with varying emphasis on these approaches (Fowler-Brown & Kahwati, 2004). Reviews and analyses of current obesity interventions indicate a range of outcomes. In general, it has proven easier to impact significant changes in healthy lifestyle behaviors versus changes in weight and BMI status. Thomas and Stern (1995), in an Institute of Health publication, recommend that outcome measure standards include improved health behaviors (e.g., increase in fruit intake, decrease in sugar intake, increase in physical activity, decreases in sedentary behaviors) and obesity-related co-morbidities.

Obtaining qualitative outcome data, such as parent satisfaction and feedback surveys, provide additional information regarding aspects of the interventions that were most helpful and not helpful. The surveys also provide more in-depth information about successes, solutions, and remaining barriers to healthy lifestyle change and maintenance. The Lean Family program survey results have contributed to our emphasis on addressing emotional and psychological factors contributing to eating behaviors and to our modifications of program structure and content in order to better meet the needs of the children and families.

Where Do We Go from Here?

This chapter has emphasized the complexities of childhood obesity, including the multiple factors that influence the etiology, prevalence, and maintenance of childhood obesity at individual and societal levels. Successful intervention with the growing childhood obesity epidemic will require multi-faceted approaches operating in immediate child–parent, family, community, and societal contexts in order to address the individual, multi-cultural, and social-ecological factors impacting childhood obesity (Ashe et al., 2007; Kitzman & Beech, 2006; Peterson & Fox, 2007). Combined efforts of families, clinicians, communities, academia, industry, governing entities, and international groups are needed to support and maintain healthy lifestyle behaviors and avoid public health pandemic (Economos & Hauser, 2007; Huang & Horlick, 2007; Peterson & Fox, 2007).

Evidence for the efficacy of clinical family-based behavioral interventions for childhood obesity has been strong and consistent (Epstein et al., 2007) with meta-analysis results indicating "large and reliable effects that also appear to be maintained across follow-up intervals spanning several months" (Young et al., 2007, p. 247). The reviewed interventions included high levels of parent involvement, and treatment components addressing dietary and physical activity behaviors through the use of psychoeducation and behavior change strategies (Young et al., 2007). Additional studies offer promise for other treatment options including variations of parent-based strategies, school-based programs, use of more intense social-cognitive strategies, use of motivational interviewing, and interventions to match change stages (Bagby & Adams, 2007; Cole et al., 2006; Golan, 2006; Epstein et al., 2007; Kitzman & Beech, 2006). Based on this body of research and direct clinical experience with the Lean Family programs at Tripler Army Medical Center, clinicians were presented practical guidelines for the development of childhood obesity programs.

Despite promising research and programs, additional study is needed to specify treatment component effects on particular outcomes; clarify the impact of combined group, separate group, family, and individual treatment formats at various child developmental levels; explore ideal levels and types of child and parent involvement at various child developmental levels; assess the efficacy and cost-benefits of additional parent intervention components (i.e., parenting, stress management, communication and coping skills); and explore the differential effects of ethnicity, SES, geography, culture, and gender with regard to these treatment variables (Germann et al., 2007; Golan, 2006; Epstein et al., 2007; Kitzman & Beech, 2006; Kumanyika, 2004). Similarly, more systematic study of relationships between child/family change stage status and treatment strategy impact can serve to maximize resources and improve efficacy of interventions (Golan, 2006).

Particular efforts should be made to promote research and development of effective obesity interventions for young ethnic minorities (particularly Black, Latino, Native American and Pacific Islander populations; Kumanyika, 2004) given differential increasing prevalence rates and a decline in efficacious interventions (Germann et al., 2007). Additional work is needed to develop effective, intensive programs to fill the gap in services for severely obese youth (Epstein et al, 2007). Also, research and development of feasible obesity preventive and early intervention strategies for younger aged children in the 2- to 5-year-old and 5- to 8-year-old age ranges are needed to combat increasing overweight status at younger ages (Epstein, 2003) and to capitalize on evidence suggesting that intervening earlier in life will lead to greater long-term behavior change success (Ahina, 2003). Adapting programs to intervene at locations with consistent and high access to young children—such as schools, afterschool programs, and primary health care settings—would help in efforts to tide rising child obesity trends (Jelalian & Mehlenbeck, 2003; Peterson & Fox, 2007).

Lastly, it is important to encourage ongoing research on the biological factors related to childhood obesity to include genetic, molecular, hormonal, and pharmacological areas of study (Epstein et al., 2007; Huang & Horlick, 2007; Jelalian & Mehlenbeck, 2003) and to incorporate this knowledge with intervention efforts.

References

Ahina, L. K. (2003). Kids Lite: A family treatment for pediatric obesity. Unpublished doctoral dissertation, Argosy University, Hawaii Campus.

Ashe, M., Feldstein, L. M., Graff, S., Kline, R., Pinkas, D., & Zellers, L. (2007). Local venues for change: Legal strategies for healthy environments. *Journal of Law, Medicine & Ethics, 35*, 138–147.

Bagby, K. & Adams, S. (2007). Evidence-based practice guideline: Increasing physical activity in schools—Kindergarten through 8th grade. *Journal of School Nursing, 23*, 137–143.

Bandura, A. (1986). *Social foundations of thought and action: A social cognitive theory.* Englewood Cliffs, NJ: Prentice Hall.

Berry, D., Savoye, M., Melkus, G., & Grey, M. (2007). An intervention for multiethnic obese parents and overweight children. *Applied Nursing Research, 20*, 63–71.

Blatner, A. (2001). Psychodrama. In R. J. Corsini (Ed.), *Handbook of innovative therapies* (2nd ed., pp. 535–545). New York: Wiley.

Bronfenbrenner, U. (1979). *The ecology of human development: Experiments by nature and design.* Cambridge, MA: Harvard University Press.

Chehab, L. G., Pfeffer, B., Vargas, I., Chen, S., & Irigoyen, M. (2007). "Energy Up": A novel approach to the weight management of inner-city teens. *Journal of Adolescent Health, 40*, 474–476.

Cole, K., Waldrop, J., D'Auria, J., & Garner, H. (2006). An integrative research review: Effective school-based childhood overweight interventions. *Journal for Specialists in Pediatric Nursing*, 11(3), 166–176.

Davis, S. P., Northington, L., & Kolar, K. (2000). Cultural considerations for treatment of childhood obesity. *Journal of Cultural Diversity, 7*, 128–132.

Drohan, S. H. (2002). Managing early childhood obesity in the primary care setting: A behavior modification approach. *Pediatric Nursing, 28*, 599–610.

Economos, C. D., & Irish-Hauser, S. (2007). Community interventions: A brief overview and their application to the obesity epidemic. *Journal of Law, Medicine & Ethics, 35*, 131–137.

Epstein, L. H. (2003). Development of evidence-based treatments for pediatric obesity. In A. E. Kazdin & J. R. Weisz (Eds.), *Evidence-based psychotherapies for children and adolescents* (pp. 374–388). New York: Guilford Press.

Epstein, L. H., Paluch, R. A., Kilanowski, C. K., & Raynor, H. A. (2004). The effect of reinforcement or stimulus control to reduce sedentary behavior in the treatment of pediatric obesity. *Healthy Psychology, 23*, 371–380.

Epstein, L. H., Paluch, R. A., Roemmich, J. N., & Beecher, M. D. (2007). Family-based obesity treatment, then and now: Twenty-five years of pediatric obesity treatment. *Health Psychology, 26*, 381–391.

Evans, H. L., & Sullivan, M. A. (1993). Children and the use of self-monitoring, self-evaluation, and self-reinforcement. In A. J. Finch, W. M. Nelson, & E. S. Ott (Eds.), *Cognitive behavioral procedures with children and adolescents* (pp. 67–89). Boston: Allyn and Bacon.

Fitzpatrick-Nietschmann, J. (1983). Pacific islanders-migration and health. *Western Journal of Medicine, Dec*, 139(6), 848–853.

Flegal, K. M., Carroll, M. D., Ogden, C. L., & Johnson, C. L. (2002). Prevalence and trends in overweight among US adults, 1999–2000. *Journal of the American Medical Association, 288*, 1723–1727.

Fowler-Brown, A., & Kahwati, L. C. (2004). Prevention and treatment of overweight in children and adolescents. *American Family Physician, 69*, 2591–2598.

Germann, J. N., Kirschenbaum, D. S., & Rich, B. H. (2006). Use of an orientation session may help decrease attrition in a pediatric weight management program for low-income minority adolescents. *Journal of Clinical Psychology in Medical Settings, 13*, 177–187.

Golan, M. (2006). Parents as agents of change in childhood obesity—From research to practice. *International Journal of Pediatric Obesity*, 1(2), 66–76.

Goldfield, G. S., Epstein, L. H., Kilanowski, C. K., Paluch, R. A., & Kogut-Bossler, B. (2001). Cost-effectiveness of group and mixed family-based treatment for childhood obesity. *International Journal of Obesity, 25*, 1843–1849.

Howard, K. R. (2007). Childhood overweight: Parental perceptions and readiness for change. *Journal of School Nursing, 23*, 73–79.

Huang, T. T., & Horlick, M. N. (2007). Trends in childhood obesity research: A brief analysis of NIH-supported efforts. *Journal of Law, Medicine & Ethics, 35*, 148–153.

James, L.C., Folen, R.A., Page, H., Noce, M. & Britton, C. (1999). The Tripler LEAN program: A two-year follow-up report. *Military Medicine, 164*, 389–395.

James, L., Folen, R. Garland, F., Noce, M., Edwards, C., Gohdes, D. et al. (1997). The Tripler LEAN PROGRAM: A healthy lifestyle model for the treatment of obesity. *Military Medicine, 162*, 328–332.

Janicke, D. M., Sallinen, B. J., Perri, M. G., Lutes, L. D., Silverstein, J. H., Huerta, M. G. et al. (2007). Sensible treatment of obesity in rural youth (STORY): Design and method. *Contemporary Clinical Trials*, doi: 10.1016/j.cct.2007.05.005.

Jelalian, E., & Mehlenbeck, R. (2003). Pediatric obesity. In M. C. Roberts (Ed.), *Handbook of pediatric psychology* (3rd ed., pp. 529–543). New York: Guilford Press.

Jelalian, E., & Saelens, B. E. (1999). Empirically supported treatments in pediatric psychology: Pediatric obesity. *Journal of Pediatric Psychology, 24*, 223–248.

Johnston, C. A., & Steele, R. G. (2007). Treatment in pediatric overweight: An examination of feasibility and effectiveness in an applied clinical setting. *Journal of Pediatric Psychology, 32*, 106–110.

Kazak, A. (1989). Families of chronically ill children: A systems and social-ecological model of adaptation and change. *Journal of Consulting and Clinical Psychology, 57*, 25–30.

Kitzmann, K. M., & Beech, B. M. (2006). Family-based interventions for pediatric obesity: Methodological and conceptual challenges from family psychology. *Journal of Family Psychology, 20*, 175–189.

Koplan, J. P., Liverman, C. T., & Kraak, V. I. (Eds.). (2005). *Preventing childhood obesity: Health in the balance*. Washington, DC: The National Academic Press.

Kumanyika, S. (2002). Obesity treatment in minorities. In T. A. Wadden, & A. J. Stunkard (Eds.), *Handbook of obesity treatment* (pp. 416–446). New York: Guilford Press.

Kumanyika, S. (2004). Cultural differences as influences on approaches to obesity treatment. In G. A. Bray, & E. Bouchard (Eds.), *Handbook of obesity: Clinical applications* (2nd ed., pp. 45–67). New York: Marcel Dekker.

Miller, W. M., & Rollnick, S. (2002). *Motivational interviewing* (2nd ed.). New York: Guilford Press.

Nguyen-Rodriguez, S.T., Chou, C.P., Unger, J.B., & Spruijt-Metz, D. (2008). BMI as a moderator of perceived stress and emotional eating in adolescents. *Eating Behaviors*, 9(2), 238–246.

Ogden, C. L., Carroll, M. D., Curtin, L. R., McDowell, M. A., Tabak, C. J., & Flegal, K. M. (2006). Prevalence of overweight and obesity in the United States, 1999–2004. *Journal of the American Medical Association*, 295, 1549–1555.

Peterson, K.E., & Fox, M.K. (2007). Addressing the epidemic of childhood obesity through school-based interventions: What has been done and where do we go from here? *Journal of Law, Medicine & Ethics*, 35, 113–130.

Piaget, J. (1962). *Play, dreams and imitation in childhood*. New York: Norton.

Prochaska, J. O., & DiClemente, C. C. (1983). Stages and processes of self-change of smoking: Toward an integrative model of change. *Journal of Consulting and Clinical Psychology*, 51, 390–395.

Prochaska, J. O., & Velicer, W. F. (1997). The transtheoretical model of health behavior change. *American Journal of Health Promotion*, 12, 38–48.

Resnicow, K., Davis, R., & Rollnick, S. (2006). Motivational interviewing for pediatric obesity: Conceptual issues and evidence review. *Journal of the American Dietetic Association*, 106, 2024–2033.

Robert Wood Johnson Foundation Newsletter. (2007, April 4). *Foundation commits $500 million to reverse childhood obesity*. Princeton, NJ. Retrieved April 4, 2008, from http://www.rwjf.org/programareas/approach.jsp?pid=1138.

Sherwood, N. E. & Jeffery, R. W. (2007). Primary prevention of obesity. In J. A. Trafton & W. P. Gordon (Eds.), *Best practices in the behavioral management of chronic disease: Vol. 1* (ch. 17, pp. 427–445). Los Altos, CA: Institute for Disease Management.

Spurlock, M. (Producer/Director). (2004). *Super Size Me* [Motion Picture]. United States: Arts Alliance America.

Thomas, P. R. & Stern, J. S. (1995). Summary. In P. R. Thomas, & J. S. Stern (Eds.), *Weighing the options: Criteria for evaluating the outcomes of approaches to prevent and treat obesity*. Washington, DC: National Academy Press.

US Department of Agriculture. (2005). *Dietary guidelines*. Retrieved May 4, 2006, from http://mypyramid.gov/guidelines/index.html.

US Department of Health and Human Services. (2001). *The Surgeon General's call to action to prevent and decrease overweight and obesity*. Washington, DC: US Department of Health and Human Services, Office of Surgeon General, Government Printing Office.

Young, K., Northern, J. J., Lister, K. M., Drummond, J. A., & O'Brien, W. (2007). A meta-analysis of family-behavioral weight-loss treatments for children. *Clinical Psychology Review*, 27, 240–249.

Chapter 3
Adolescent Obesity: Review of the Treatment Literature

Valerie H. Myers and Brooke L. Barbera

Introduction

Childhood and adolescent obesity is a worldwide health concern due to its rapidly increasing prevalence and its associated medical and social consequences (Fowler-Brown, & Kahwati, 2004). The number of overweight children in the United States is reaching epidemic proportions. The Centers for Disease Control and Prevention (CDC) classify overweight in children and adolescents according to two levels: (1) being at risk for overweight, which is identified as a body mass index (BMI) between the 85th and 95th percentiles for age and gender as measured by growth charts from the National Center for Health Statistics for children aged 2–17 and (2) being overweight, which is determined by a BMI of 95th percentile for age and gender (Kuczmarski et al., 2002; Ogden et al., 2006). The prevalence of obesity in children and adolescents is higher than 20 years ago in all ethnic, age, and gender groups, and obesity among teenagers has nearly tripled (Hedley et al., 2004; Ogden, Flegal, Carroll, & Johnson, 2002). The most recent National Health and Nutrition Examination Survey (NHANES) revealed that 34.3% of adolescents between the ages of 12 and 19 years are overweight or at risk for becoming overweight (Ogden et al., 2006). Currently, over 10 million children in the United States are at risk for overweight, and children are becoming obese at younger ages. Estimates suggest that 80% of overweight 10- to 15-year-olds will become obese adults if successful interventions are not developed (Hill & Throwbridge, 1998). Several risk factors for excess weight in children have been identified including gender, race/ethnicity, socioeconomic status, and obese parents. Notably, adolescent obesity often originates during the early childhood years and is persistent and difficult to treat.

Consequences of Obesity

The escalating rates of adolescent obesity will impact the future health of Americans. Overweight adolescents have a 70% chance of becoming overweight or obese adults (U.S. Department of Health and Human Services, 2007), and the impact of adolescent overweight continues into adulthood (Fowler-Brown & Kahwati, 2004). There are a number of serious medical complications and risk factors associated with child obesity, many of which typically occur only in adult populations. Pediatric obesity is a serious

V.H. Myers (✉)
Pennington Biomedical Research Center, Louisiana State University System, Baton Rouge, LA, USA
e-mail: valerie.myers@pbrc.edu

L.C. James, J.C. Linton (eds.), *Handbook of Obesity Intervention for the Lifespan*,
DOI 10.1007/978-0-387-78305-5_4, © Springer Science+Business Media, LLC 2009

chronic disease that contributes to conditions such as hypertension, hypercholesterole-
mia, diabetes, glucose intolerance, some forms of cancer, and increased musculoskeletal
injuries (American Academy of Pediatrics Committee on Nutrition, 2003). Other consequences of childhood obesity include advanced maturation. Obese children have
advanced bone age, higher bone density and area, and increased sexual hormone levels
(De Simone et al., 1995). In addition to the physical sequelae of childhood obesity,
research indicates that psychosocial problems are a serious and prevalent long-term
consequence of childhood obesity (Hill & Throwbridge, 1998). Obese children may
experience lowered self-esteem and increased depression ratings as well as discrimination
by peers, family members, and teachers. Notably, in a recent study, self-reported quality
of life of severely overweight children was five times lower than normal-weight children
and was remarkably equal to that reported by children with terminal cancer (Schwimmer,
Burwinkle, & Varni, 2003).

Causes of Obesity

Obesity is a disorder of energy balance, in which the number of calories consumed exceeds
the number of calories expended. Obesity results when susceptible (i.e., genetically predisposed) individuals are exposed to obesity-promoting environments (Hill & Throwbridge,
1998). According to the U.S. Surgeon General, the causes of overweight in children can be
categorized into several factors including the following: (1) a lack of physical activity,
unhealthy eating patterns, or a combination of the two, with genetics and lifestyle both
playing important roles, (2) an increase in sedentary behaviors in our society, that is,
television and computer and video games, contribute to children's inactive lifestyles, and
(3) children, especially girls, become less active as they move through adolescence (U.S.
Department of Health and Human Services, 2007). According to the current scientific
literature, definitive causes of overweight condition in childhood still remain unclear. However, there is evidence that weight and adiposity are entrained during early life (Dietz, 1994).
Research suggests that familial factors impact the development of childhood obesity. However, it remains unclear as to what extent genetics and environment impact on these familial
factors. Parental obesity is the single most important predictor of adult obesity in children
under the age of 10 years (Whitaker, Wright, Pepe, Seidel, & Dietz, 1997). Estimates suggest
that only 7% of children will become obese when born to normal-weight parents. The risk of
childhood obesity increases to 40% when one parent is obese, and when both parents are
obese the risk becomes 80%. Genetics plays an important role; however, family environment
has the greatest impact on a child's weight (Dietz & Gortmaker, 2001). Notably, as a child
matures, his/her weight becomes a stronger predictor of adult obesity.

Despite the increase in pediatric obesity over the past decades, there remains a dearth of
evidence for efficacious treatments in this population. There are only a handful of peer-
reviewed, vigorously designed studies on pediatric obesity, the majority of which have
focused on school-aged children under the age of 12 years. Little empirical evidence exists
for validated treatments with adolescents. The existing treatment literature focuses on
implementing the two key components to the treatment of overweight in children and
adolescents – the introduction of healthy dietary intake and increased physical activity.
Fortunately, both of these factors are behavioral in nature and are therefore modifiable.
The modification of dietary intake and physical activity among children and adolescents
has been reported in a number of treatment settings. In addition to these two target areas,

another key component to treatment with children and adolescents is the use of behavior modification. Behavioral strategies found to be most effective in reduction of weight include goal setting, self-monitoring, stimulus control, contingency management, social reinforcement, relapse prevention, and problem solving. A full review of behavior modification techniques in detail would be beyond the scope of this chapter. The primary aim of this chapter is to highlight the intervention literature for adolescents in the following areas: school and Internet, family, primary care, and multi-component (i.e., combination of more than one area). The focus of the review will be on randomized controlled trials.

School-Based and Internet-Based Interventions

Children and adolescents spend a majority of their daily hours in the school environment. Given the educational mission of these institutions, schools are key settings for targeting behavior change and teaching lifelong health practices. School-based interventions have the potential to introduce and establish healthy eating and exercise patterns that may persist into adulthood (Lytle, Seifert, Greenstein, & McGovern, 2000). A great amount of research literature describes multiple behavior interventions as the key for both obesity prevention and treatment. Indeed, interventions in school settings can focus on a wide range of behaviors, including increasing physical activity, limiting sedentary behaviors (i.e., television viewing), improving the nutritional quality of both school meals and available snack foods, increasing fruit and vegetable consumption, and teaching students about long-term healthy eating and exercise behaviors. School programs targeted at obesity in adolescents can also involve parents to help make changes at home.

The emphasis of the literature regarding school-based interventions for children is on making healthy decisions as early as possible in children's lives. The school-based literature for adolescents over the age of 12 is markedly limited, with more focus on identifiable changes in the school environment or the modification of behaviors in a model similar to adult interventions that focus on multi-component lifestyle change. The participants in these studies are not limited to already overweight students, as earlier research shows that targeting only those students can provoke teasing (Story, 1999). Results of these interventions are mixed. In several studies, the interventions successfully prevented an increase in BMI in primarily female students and increased physical activity and nutrition knowledge in both genders. Notably, many published school-based intervention studies did not evaluate weight gain as the main variable of interest and were designed primarily to observe changes in cardiovascular health, nutritional intake and/or knowledge, or physical activity patterns. Many interventions were theory driven, based on social cognitive theory, Pender's health promotion model, or the transtheoretical model, thus focusing more on process variables of self-efficacy or readiness to change behaviors instead of actual weight change.

Two efficacious studies with theory-driven models include the New Moves Prevention Program (Neumark-Sztainer, Story, Hannan, & Rex, 2003), which offered an alternative form of physical education to high-school girls and included information on social support and nutrition to physical activity. The intervention group showed no significant changes in BMI as compared with the control. However, authors reported a significantly greater progression of stages of change for physical activity postintervention (31% for intervention schools, 20% for control schools). At follow-up, 38% of the intervention participants had progressed and 11% regressed, while the control participants remained unchanged in their readiness to change physical activity behavior. An important implication of these results is that female-only tailored physical education classes may be one avenue to increase exercise behaviors in girls who perceive barriers in traditional co-ed classes. A slightly smaller, less intensive intervention with 6th through 8th graders by Frenn, Malin, and Bansal (2003) demonstrated that additional, tailored classroom sessions could have a positive impact on exercise duration, with greater duration of exercise in the intervention group. Frenn and colleagues also reported that the percentage of fat intake was significantly lower in the group receiving specialized classroom sessions.

Some of the most promising interventions use a combination of techniques and modes of treatment, working toward a model of making health-conscious lifestyle choices rather than singular behavior change. These interventions have the common focus of promoting a healthy weight rather than losing weight (Barlow & Dietz, 1998). Planet Health was a 2-year intervention study of over 1000 middle-school students (assessed during grades 6–9) across 48 schools that incorporated healthy eating and fitness lessons into several courses across disciplines (language, math, science, social studies, physical education) (Gortmaker et al., 1999). This program was innovative in its combination of cognitive (i.e., social cognitive theory) and behavioral elements, in addition to changing environmental aspects (e.g., food service staff education, kitchen equipment improvements), parent education, and the creation of student health committees. Girls in the intervention schools showed improved change in obesity prevalence and fruit and vegetable intake but did not increase physical activity. Boys showed improved BMIs and showed significant improvements in physical activity levels. In both genders, the level of television viewing was reduced in intervention schools. Researchers investigating and implementing this program completed an economic analysis of this broad-range, multi-component intervention and found it to be cost-effective for schools (Wang, Yang, Lowry, & Weschler, 2003).

Research trials such as Health in Motion (Mauriello et al., 2006) and Health Improvement Program for Teens (HIP Teens) (White et al., 2004; Williamson, Martin, White, Newton, & Walden, 2003) have also incorporated the use of computers and Internet access in the school environment for assessment, education, and intervention. The Health in Motion effectiveness trial began in September 2006 in eight high schools. Its focus is healthy lifestyle choices for all students regardless of weight. Based on the transtheoretical model, a primary outcome is the progression of students through stages of change for the target health behaviors: decreased sedentary behavior through television viewing, increased fruit and vegetable consumption, and increased physical activity. The program was pilot tested with 45 participants in 11th and 12th grades and demonstrated the feasibility of applying a computer-based education tool into one or several classroom sessions. The computer program is interactive, includes both assessments of and feedback on the target behaviors, and incorporates narratives from other high-school students. Results of the Health in Motion trial are pending, but the authors relate programs like this to computer-based bullying prevention programs that have documented effectiveness and are now marketed to schools across the United States (Mauriello et al.). The HIP Teens Project applied an Internet-based behavioral weight loss intervention to overweight and obese African-American girls, aged 11–15 years, and to their parents (White et al., 2004; Williamson et al., 2003, 2006). Building on research indicating behavioral interventions as superior to primarily educational programs, the behavioral intervention utilized email communication with a case manager specially trained in weight management. The core of the program was a website that presented behavioral-aimed weekly topics (e.g., goal setting, problem solving, self-monitoring), provided the automated form participants used to log food records, and provided health information for parent–child dyads (Williamson et al., 2003). Behavioral groups were also conducted, and participants set physical activity goals with their case manager and peers. The results of HIP Teens were decreased body fat for adolescent girls and decreased body weight in their parents after 6 months of treatment, but these changes were not maintained at 18 months. Self-reported levels of exercise for girls and parents were associated with greater weight and fat loss at 24 months. Website tracking of log-ins showed that website use decreased significantly after the first study year (Williamson et al., 2006).

In summary, school environments can be a positive arena for the promotion of healthy food choices and increased opportunities for physical activity. Some environmental recommendations are becoming a practice, as public officials in Philadelphia, Pennsylvania, recently passed a law prohibiting vending machines in public schools. Other schools are following suit, also discouraging unhealthy food (pizza party, donut day, etc.) as rewards for good behavior or academic accomplishment. These small environmental changes are positive, but the above research suggests more ecological changes are needed, and behavioral interventions should be promoted. Continued research into adolescent-targeted interventions is needed to better understand the impact of weight management for adolescents and young adults who may or may not learned healthy weight practices at younger ages.

Family-Based and Individual Interventions

Interventions for overweight children and adolescents often use family-based counseling approaches. Family behavioral counseling and parent training are effective methods for the prevention and treatment of pediatric obesity and are a critical component of treatment studies that have shown efficacious results. The research suggests that a family therapy component to treatment (e.g., the child and a minimum of one parent receiving instruction) results in significant reductions in overweight. Unfortunately, few controlled studies using a family-based focus have utilized adolescents only (e.g., children between the ages of 12 and 17 years). Notable efficacious studies include Brownell, Kelman, and Stunkard (1983) who reported significantly greater weight loss in youth between the ages of 12 and 16 years who participated in counseling separate from parents, compared to those youth treated alone or in tandem with their parent. In this study, the mother and youth were either (1) treated separately (both attended separate groups), (2) treated together (mother and youth attended the same group), or (3) youth treated alone. The mother–youth group of adolescents treated separately lost more weight during treatment compared with the two other conditions, and differences between the groups increased at a 1-year follow-up. These findings suggest that parental involvement is a critical component, but perhaps some amount of autonomy for the youth is equally important. In a second study of adolescents, Wadden and colleagues (1990) examined a behavioral weight control program in overweight African-American females. All of the youth participated in the same 16-week weight loss program, but the girls differed in the amount of parental involvement they had. Specifically, the youth were treated alone, in combination with mother, or treated separately. Youth in all three treatment conditions lost weight; however, there were no statistical differences between the groups. A notable finding was that youth lost more weight with the greater number of sessions attended by the mother. This suggests that parental involvement plays a role in the weight loss success of adolescents; however, the amount and extent of that involvement remains unclear. Another randomized study illustrated that parent participation enhanced the weight loss of adolescents enrolled in a group multidisciplinary weight loss program that included calorie restriction, exercise, and behavioral counseling (Coates, Kilien, & Slinkard, 1982). The study incorporated parent or no-parent participation. Parents in the participation group received learning skills for assisting in their child's weight loss. Adolescents in the parent participation condition produced greater weight loss results at 15 weeks. Unfortunately, the findings were not maintained, and by 9 months, weight loss was similar between the parent and no-parent participation groups with no statistical differences. Another study, SHAPEDOWN, was an adolescent obesity intervention with a randomized experimental design (Mellin, Slinkard, & Irwin, 1987). Test groups were compared with no-treatment controls, and the active program included cognitive behavioral techniques to make small modifications in diet and exercise. Parents were instructed on strategies to support their child's weight loss efforts. Significant improvements in weight at posttreatment and 1-year follow-up were found for those adolescents participating in the treatment group.

There are a number of other controlled and effectiveness trials with adolescents that have resulted in notable findings. Ebbeling, Leidig, Sinclair, Hangen, and Ludwig (2003) conducted a study indicating that low-glycemic (LG) diets may promote significantly greater improvements in the metabolic profiles of sedentary, overweight adolescents when compared with balanced calorie meal plans. Rocchini et al. (1988) and Becque, Katch, Rocchini, Marks, and Moorehead (1988) noted reductions in percentage of fat among adolescents receiving 20 weeks of treatment focused on diet, exercise, and behavior change. In addition, there are a number of studies that have included adolescents; however, children under the age of 12 were also included in the study. The majority of these studies contained several common elements – a combination of diet, exercise/physical activity, and behavior modification. These studies demonstrated that the inclusion of the family in counseling sessions improved both short-term and long-term outcomes with similar findings across studies. A more comprehensive list of family-based and individual randomized clinical trials in children and adolescents is available (Myers & Martin, 2006).

In summary, behavioral counseling for weight reduction in adolescents has been shown to be an effective method for modifying dietary and exercise patterns. The common components of diet, physical activity, and behavior modification have been shown to be the standards of success among efficacious studies of youth. However, it should be noted that family-based and long-term studies in adolescents are lacking compared to studies in children under the age of 12 years. There is mixed evidence regarding the benefits of group, family-based counseling with adolescents. It remains unclear whether adolescents would benefit more from behavioral counseling alone or with parents. Large-scale, randomized clinical trials focusing on tailored, age-appropriate messages of weight reduction and healthy lifestyle for adolescents are still needed.

Primary-Care Interventions

Prevention and treatment is the cornerstone of pediatric practice. With the increasing trend of overweight and obesity among children, the primary-care setting has become a logical setting for combating the obesity epidemic (American Academy of Pediatrics Committee on Nutrition, 2003), and the pediatrician plays an important role in the prevention of childhood obesity. Unfortunately, the potential role of prevention and treatment through primary care is currently under-rated by the medical community. According to the U.S. Surgeon General (U.S. Department of Health and Human Services, 2007), the determination of overweight in children and adolescents should adhere to the following guidelines: (1) physicians and other health-care professionals are the most qualified people to determine whether a child's weight is unhealthy, (2) BMI should be calculated from measurements of height and weight with the use of a BMI growth chart, and (3) a physician will also consider the child's age and growth patterns to determine whether his or her weight is healthy. Given that the primary-care setting is the recommended source for identifying overweight among children, it is a logical setting for intervention. Additionally, clinically overweight or obese children are presenting with more chronic disease risk factors, and the physician delivers treatment of these diseases in a comprehensive manner. Clinical pediatric obesity interventions should be delivered by a team of health-care experts in a medically supervised, nurturing, and non-intimidating environment. Unfortunately, despite the primary-care setting as an opportune location for weight loss programs, physician-based interventions that provide vital nutrition and physical activity education, including parenting skills, are still desperately needed.

Few clinical trials have evaluated the use of behavioral weight loss programs for overweight adolescents. Saelens and colleagues (2002) evaluated the posttreatment and short-term follow-up efficacy of a 4-month behavioral weight control program for overweight adolescents in a primary-care setting. The results indicated that a physician-based, individual counseling program including nutrition and physical activity education was superior to a standard care approach in overweight teenagers. Dreimane and colleagues (2007) examined the feasibility of a hospital-based, family-centered intervention (Kids N Fitness) targeting overweight children and adolescents between the ages of 7 and 17 years. This program consisted of interactive nutrition and physical activity sessions with behavior modification in an outpatient setting. Results showed that weight and BMI were lower during the behavioral program compared with those children in the pre-program observation period. In another hospital-based study of morbidly obese, low-income minority adolescents (the La Rabida Children's Hospital FitMatters Program), participants received cognitive behavioral therapy, nutrition education, structured exercise, and medical monitoring (Germann, Kirschenbaum, Rich, & O'Koon, 2006). About a quarter of the participants achieved a clinically meaningful weight change at 2 years. Analyses revealed that successful participants compared with less-successful participants attended more treatment sessions and utilized more critical weight loss skills (e.g., self-monitoring). Another robust, randomized trial that combined the resources of the primary-care clinic in conjunction with home-based strategies compared a comprehensive multimodal approach to a comparison control (Patrick et al., 2006). Participants in the experimental condition received primary care, office-based, computer-assisted diet and physical activity assessment with brief health-care provider counseling. Additionally, the participants received 1 year of monthly counseling by telephone and postal mail contact. Measures of physical activity and changes in dietary intake were the primary outcomes. BMI was a secondary outcome. Adolescents in the experimental condition significantly reduced sedentary behavior compared to those in the control condition. Trends were seen toward improvements in dietary intake. Unfortunately, changes in BMI did not reach statistical significance. These findings suggest that although reducing sedentary behavior is important in the overall health of adolescents, changes in diet in order to produce significant changes in weight is still needed.

Pharmacotherapy

There have been only a limited number of trials exploring the use of pharmacotherapy in pediatric obesity treatment, and its use in adolescents remains a controversial topic. In general, only adolescents with a BMI greater than the 95th percentile or higher for their age and gender plus an obesity-related medical condition should be considered for pharmacotherapy (Yanovski & Yanovski, 2002). There are two drugs currently available for the long-term treatment of overweight conditions during adolescence – orlistat (a gastric and pancreatic inhibitor) and sibutramine (norepinephrine-serotonin reuptake inhibitor).

Berkowitz, Wadden, Tershakovec, and Cronquist (2003) observed a synergistic effect of adding sibutramine to a multi-disciplinary behavioral weight loss treatment intervention in adolescents. This randomized, double-blind, placebo-controlled trial examined whether additional weight loss was achieved in obese adolescence when sibutramine was added to a family-based, behavioral weight control program. The results showed that participants in the behavior therapy and sibutramine group lost significantly more weight than those in the behavior therapy and placebo condition. In a follow-up study, these trends were repeated when comparing African-American and Caucasian adolescents (Budd et al., 2007). Sibutramine impacted reductions in weight loss in both African-American and Caucasian teens. In another clinical trial of sibutramine, Godoy-Matos and colleagues (2005) examined the efficacy and safety of sibutramine in obese adolescents. This trial was a randomized, double-blind, placebo-controlled trial. All participants received placebo and a hypocaloric diet plus exercise for the first month of the study. For the next 6 months, participants received either sibutramine or placebo. Participants receiving sibutramine group lost significantly more weight and had greater BMI reduction than those on placebo.

McDuffie and colleagues (2002) examined the 3-month safety, tolerability, and efficacy of orlistat in obese adolescents. Participants received 3 months of orlistat and a multivitamin as well as a 12-week behavioral program emphasizing diet, exercise, and strategies for behavior change. The results revealed that weight and BMI decreased significantly. In another study to determine the effects of orlistat compared to placebo, Chanoine, Hampl, Jensen, Boldrin, and Hauptman (2005) investigated the effect of orlistat on weight and body composition in obese adolescents. This trial was a multi-center, randomized, double-blind study of a 120-mg dose of orlistat or placebo. Both treatment conditions received a mildly hypocaloric diet, physical activity, and behavioral therapy. Both treatment groups displayed a reduction in BMI up to 12 weeks. At the end of the study, there was a significant difference between BMI in the orlistat and control group, with the orlistat group experiencing better weight outcomes. However, both treatment groups experienced weight regain at study end. In another study of orlistat (Ozkan, Bereket, Turan, & Keskin, 2004), obese adolescents were given orlistat in combination with a nutritional and lifestyle intervention. The comparison group received conventional treatment alone (no behavioral treatment). Adolescents in the orlistat plus behavior therapy condition reported significantly more weight loss than those adolescents receiving conventional treatment. Notably, a third of the adolescents in the orlistat group dropped out of the study within the first month due to side effects of the medication.

Although the use of weight loss medication for weight loss in adolescents seems promising, published clinical trial data is limited. It is important to note that there are side effects associated with medication use, such as increase in blood pressure with sibutramine and gastrointestinal disturbance with orlistat. The clinical trial data that is available has shown the efficacy of these drugs; however, all of the trials have used behavioral weight control programs in combination with the medication. There is no stand-alone data for the use of the medications for weight loss, and until these data are available, medications should be limited to settings that provide comprehensive treatment for obese adolescents.

Surgery in Adolescents

Surgery as a method of treatment has been an option for adults for over four decades. A comprehensive history on the development of the various surgical techniques is beyond the scope of this chapter (Sjostrom, 2000). There are two broad classifications of weight loss surgeries – restrictive procedures and restrictive procedures with malabsorption. Restrictive procedures reduce the size of the stomach pouch, whereas restrictive-malabsorptive procedures combine a restrictive procedure with a partial bypass of the small intestine. Both methods results in weight loss by decreasing the daily caloric intake of the individual.

There is a dearth of data on the impact of adolescent bariatric treatments, and the majority of studies on this topic are retrospective in nature. Bariatric surgery for adolescents has not been formerly recommended due to the lack of sufficient data on the topic. Nonetheless, adolescents with clinically severe obesity have been provided surgery as a viable treatment option. In an early study, Rand and Macgregor (1994) interviewed 34 adolescents aged 11–19 years 6 years postsurgery. Fifty percent weight loss was reported in 73% of patients, and average weight regain was 9 kg. The mean age at time of surgery was 17 years. Growth rate appeared unaffected, and health and psychosocial improvements were reported by most. Only 13% reported taking nutritional supplements as prescribed, and adherence to exercise and dietary recommendations was poor. In another study, follow-up data on gastric bypass outcome was evaluated among 10 adolescents (Strauss, Bradley, & Brolin, 2001). Mean weight loss was 53.6 kg. Postoperative recovery was uneventful in all adolescents, and micronutrient deficiency was the most commonly reported late complication. The authors concluded that bariatric surgery is well tolerated in adolescence and produces similar results as in adulthood. Dolan, Creighton, Hopkins, and Fielding (2003) prospectively collected data since 1996 on adolescents who received laparoscopic adjustable gastric banding (LAGB). Mean age at time of surgery was 17 years. Complications were experienced in two of the patients (i.e., a leaking port and slipped band). Over 75% of patients lost a minimum of 50% of their excess weight. The authors reported that LAGB is a safe and effective treatment for severely obese adolescents and may be a preferred method in this population, given that the procedure is reversible. In another study, the authors reviewed a 20-year-old database on bariatric surgery in adolescents (Sugerman et al., 2003). Of the 33 adolescents in the registry from 1981 to 2001, mean age at time of surgery was 16 years. Follow-up at 14 years found that 61% of excess weight lost was maintained. No operative deaths were reported; however, two patients died 2 years and 6 years postoperatively due to conditions unrelated to the surgery. Early and late complications, as well as revisional surgeries, approximated the prevalence found in the adult literature. Five of the patients had regained all weight by 10 years postoperation; however, significant weight loss was maintained in the majority up to 14 years. Garcia, Langford, and Inge (2003) reviewed the application of laparoscopic surgery in adolescents. They reported that no prospective, randomized studies comparing the efficacy of bariatric surgery to other conventional methods have been conducted. The authors encouraged the use of behavioral management programs if surgery was going to be utilized. The authors also addressed the need for systematic data to evaluate the uses of RYGB versus adjustable gastric band in this population. Specifically, adjustable gastric bands require no partitioning of the stomach, thus reducing nutritional deficits; are reversible; and can be adjusted for times of pregnancy. However, the short- and long-term weight loss with the gastric banding is not as promising, and the deterrent to developing maladaptive eating patterns is not as present as with the gastric bypass procedure. Yitzhak, Mizrahi, and Avinoach (2006) examined medical records for 60 adolescents who received laparoscopic gastric banding and were at least 3 years postoperative. Mean age at time of surgery was 16 years (9–18). Mean preoperative BMI was 43 kg/m², and mean postoperative BMI after 3 years was 30 kg/m². Six patients underwent band repositioning, and two patients underwent band removal. Dillard and colleagues (2007) evaluated weight loss efficacy and safety of LAGB in morbidly obese adolescents. The authors retrospectively reviewed data from 24 patients between the ages of 14 and 20 years. No mortality was reported. Average excess weight loss rates were 22% at 3 months, 34% at 6 months, 52% at 1 year, and 42% at 2 and 3 years. The complication rate was 29%. The authors concluded that LAGB is an effective and safe surgical weight loss method for adolescence. Notably, the authors reported that follow-up for surgery-related complications and intensive behavioral management is critical for long-term success.

Despite the encouraging results of these studies, they are retrospective in nature and represent adolescents at the extreme continuum of obesity. Systematic studies of the risks and efficacy for bariatric procedures and more conservative treatment methods in both adults and adolescents are still needed. Head-to-head comparisons of various surgical procedures and more traditional forms of treatment are lacking. The majority of data on these procedures are limited by the use of convenience samples, and there are no standardized protocols to compare study findings with one another.

Conclusion

The increasing prevalence of childhood obesity is a worldwide health concern. Adolescent obesity, which often originates during the early childhood years, is persistent and difficult to manage. Notably, a majority of teenagers will become obese adults if successful interventions are not developed. The primary goal for the treatment of pediatric obesity is healthy eating and increasing physical activity. The use of behavioral strategies in combination with dietary and physical activity improvements appear to be the critical approaches to treatment. The number of robust clinical trials targeting weight reduction in adolescents is scarce. However, research indicates that weight loss during childhood can be maintained into adulthood. Several intervention strategies and settings, including school/Internet, family, primary care, and multi-component, have shown modest success with adiposity reduction in teens. Unfortunately, the number of clinical trials focused only on adolescents remains under-investigated.

References

American Academy of Pediatrics Committee on Nutrition. (2003). Policy statement: Prevention of pediatric overweight and obesity. *Pediatrics, 112*(2), 424–430.
Barlow, S. E., & Dietz, W. H. (1998). Obesity evaluation and treatment: Expert committee recommendations. *Pediatrics, 102*(3), e29.
Becque, M. D., Katch, V. L., Rocchini, A. P., Marks, C. R., & Moorehead, C. (1988). Coronary risk incidence of obese adolescents: Reduction by exercise plus diet intervention. *Pediatrics, 81*(5), 605–612.
Berkowitz, R. I., Wadden, T. A., Tershakovec, A. M., & Cronquist, J. L. (2003). Behavior therapy and sibutramine for the treatment of adolescent obesity: A randomized controlled trial. *JAMA, 289*(14), 1805–1812.
Brownell, K. D., Kelman, J. H., & Stunkard, A. J. (1983). Treatment of obese children with and without their mothers: Changes in weight and blood pressure. *Pediatrics, 71*(4), 515–523.

Budd, G. M., Hayman, L. L., Crump, E., Pollydore, C., Hawley, K. D., Cronquist, J. L., et al. (2007). Weight loss in obese African American and Caucasian adolescents. *Journal of Cardiovascular Nursing*, *22*(4), 288–296.

Chanoine, J., Hampl, S., Jensen, C., Boldrin, M., & Hauptman, J. (2005). Effect of orlistat on weight and body composition in obese adolescents: A randomized controlled trial. *JAMA*, *293*(23), 2873–2883.

Coates, T. J., Kilien, J. D., & Slinkard, L. (1982). Parent participation in a treatment program for overweight adolescents. *International Journal of Eating Disorders*, *1*(3), 37–48.

De Simone, M., Farello, G., Palumbo, M., Gentile, T., Ciuffreda, M., Olioso, P., et al. (1995). Growth charts, growth velocity and bone development in childhood obesity. *International Journal of Obesity and Related Metabolic Disorders*, *19*(12), 851–857.

Dietz, W. H. (1994). Critical periods in childhood for the development of obesity. *American Journal of Clinical Nutrition*, *59*(5), 955–959.

Dietz, W. H., & Gortmaker, S. L. (2001). Preventing obesity in children and adolescents. *Annual Review of Public Health*, *22*: 337–353.

Dillard, B. E. 3rd, Gorodner, V., Galvani, C., Holterman, M., Browne, A., Gallo, A., et al. (2007). Initial experience with the adjustable gastric band in morbidly obese U.S. adolescents and recommendations for further investigation. *Journal of Pediatric Gastroenterology and Nutrition*, *45*(2), 240–246.

Dolan, K., Creighton, L., Hopkins, G., & Fielding, G. (2003). Laparoscopic gastric banding in morbidly obese adolescents. *Obesity Surgery*, *13*(1), 101–104.

Dreimane, D., Safani, D., MacKenzie, M., Halvorson, M., Braun, S., Conrad, B., et al. (2007). Feasibility of a hospital-based, family-centered intervention to reduce weight gain in overweight children and adolescents. *Diabetes Research & Clinical Practice*, *75*(2), 159–168.

Ebbeling, C. B., Leidig, M. M., Sinclair, K. B., Hangen, J. P., & Ludwig, D. S. (2003). A reduced-glycemic load diet in the treatment of adolescent obesity. *Archives of Pediatrics & Adolescent Medicine*, *157*(8), 773–779.

Fowler-Brown, A., & Kahwati, L. (2004). Prevention and treatment of overweight in children and adolescents. *American Family Physician*, *69*(11), 2591–2598.

Frenn, M., Malin, S., & Bansal, N. K. (2003). Stage based interventions for low-fat diet with middle school students. *Journal of Pediatric Nursing*, *18*: 36–45.

Garcia, V. F., Langford, L., & Inge, T. H. (2003). Application of laparoscopy for bariatric surgery in adolescents. *Current Opinions in Pediatrics*, *15*(3), 248–255.

Germann, J. N., Kirschenbaum, D. S., Rich, B. H., & O'Koon, J. C. (2006). Long-term evaluation of multi-disciplinary treatment of morbid obesity in low-income minority adolescents: La Rabida Children's Hospital's FitMatters program. *Journal of Adolescent Health*, *39*(4), 553–561.

Godoy-Matos, A., Carraro, L., Vieira, A., Oliveira, J., Guedes, E. P., Mattos, L., et al. (2005). Treatment of obese adolescents with sibutramine: A randomized, double blind, controlled study. *Journal of Clinical Endocrinolology & Metabolism*, *90*(3), 1460–1465.

Gortmaker, S. L., Peterson, K., Wiecha, J., Sobol, A. M., Dixit, S., Fox, M. K., et al. (1999). Reducing obesity via school-based interdisciplinary intervention among youth: Planet Health. *Archives of Pediatrics & Adolescent Medicine*, *153*, 409–418.

Hedley, A. A., Ogden, C. L., Johnson, C. L., Carroll, M. D., Curtin, L. R., & Flegal, K. M. (2004). Prevalence of overweight and obesity among US children, adolescents, and adults, 1999–2002. *JAMA*, *291*(23), 2847–2850.

Hill, J., & Throwbridge, F. (1998). The causes and health consequences of obesity in children and adolescents. *Pediatrics*, *101*(3), 497–575.

Kuczmarski, R. J., Ogden, C. L., Guo, S. S., Grummer-Strawn, L. M., Flegal, K. M., Mei, Z., et al. (2002). 2000 CDC growth charts for the United States: Methods and development. *Vital and Health Statistics*. Series 11, Data from the National Health Survey, *246*, 1–190.

Lytle, L. A., Seifert, S., Greenstein, J., & McGovern, P. (2000). How do children's eating patterns and food choices change over time? Results from a cohort study. *American Journal of Health Promotion*, *14*: 222–228.

Mauriello, L. M., Driskell, M. M., Sherman, K. J., Johnson, S. S., Prochaska, J. M., & Prochaska, J. O. (2006). Acceptability of a school-based intervention for the prevention of adolescent obesity. *The Journal of School Nursing*, *22*(5), 269–277.

McDuffie, J. R., Calis, K. A., Uwaifo, G. I., Sebring, N. G., Fallon, E. M., Hubbard, V. S., et al. (2002). Three-month tolerability of orlistat in adolescents with obesity-related comorbid conditions. *Obesity Research*, *10*(7), 642–650.

Mellin, L. M., Slinkard, L. A., & Irwin, C. E. (1987). Adolescent obesity intervention: Validation of the SHAPEDOWN program. *Journal of the American Dietetic Association, 87*(3), 333–338.

Myers, V. H., & Martin, P. D. (2006). Behavioral counseling: Family-based behavioral counseling in clinical settings. In: M. Sothern, S. T. Gordon, & T. K. von Almen (Eds.), *Handbook of pediatric obesity: Clinical management* (pp. 147–170). Boca Raton, FL: Taylor & Francis.

Neumark-Sztainer, D., Story, M., Hannan, P. J., & Rex, J. (2003). New moves: A school-based obesity prevention program for adolescent girls. *Preventive Medicine, 37*, 41–51.

Ogden, C. L., Carroll, M. D., Curtin, L. R., McDowell, M. A., Tabak, C. J., & Flegal, K. M. (2006). Prevalence of overweight and obesity in the United States, 1999–2004. *JAMA, 295*(13), 1549–1555.

Ogden, C. L., Flegal, K. M., Carroll, M. D., & Johnson, C. L. (2002). Prevalence and trends in overweight among US children and adolescents, 1999–2000. *JAMA, 288*(14), 1728.

Ozkan, B., Bereket, A., Turan, S., & Keskin, S. (2004). Addition of orlistat to conventional treatment in adolescents with severe obesity. *European Journal of Pediatrics, 163*(12), 738–741.

Patrick, K., Calfas, K. J., Norman, G. J., Zabinski, M. F., Sallis, J. F., Rupp, J., et al. (2006). Randomized controlled trial of a primary care and home-based intervention for physical activity and nutrition behaviors: PACE+ for adolescents. *Archives of Pediatrics & Adolescent Medicine, 160*(2), 128–136.

Rand, C., & Macgregor, A. (1994). Adolescents having obesity surgery: A 6-year follow-up. *Southern Medical Journal, 87*(12), 1208–1213.

Rocchini, A. P., Katch, V., Anderson, J., Hinderliter, J., Becque, M. D., Martin, M., et al. (1988). Blood pressure in obese adolescents: Effect of weight loss. *Pediatrics, 82*(1), 16–23.

Saelens, B. E., Sallis, J. F., Wilfley, D. E., Patrick, K., Cella, J. A., & Buchta, R. (2002). Behavioral weight control for overweight adolescents initiated in primary care. *Obesity Research, 10*(1), 22–32.

Schwimmer, J. B., Burwinkle, T. M., & Varni, J. W. (2003). Health-related quality of life of severely obese children and adolescents. *JAMA, 289*(14), 1813–1819.

Sjostrom, L. (2000). Surgical intervention as a strategy for treatment of obesity. *Endocrine, 13*(2), 213–230.

Story, M. (1999). School-based approaches for preventing and treating obesity. *International Journal of Obesity, 23*: S2-43–S2-51.

Strauss, R. S., Bradley, L. J., & Brolin, R. E. (2001). Gastric bypass surgery in adolescents with morbid obesity. *Journal of Pediatrics, 138*(4), 499–504.

Sugerman, H. J., Sugerman, E. L., DeMaria, E. J., Kellum, J. M., Kennedy, C., Mowery, Y., et al. (2003). Bariatric surgery for severely obese adolescents. *Journal of Gastrointestinal Surgery, 7*(1), 102–107.

U.S. Department of Health and Human Services. (2007). *The surgeon general's call to action to prevent and decrease overweight and obesity: overweight in children and adolescents*. Retrieved December 1, 2007, from USDHH website: http://www.surgeongeneral.gov/topics/obesity/calltoaction/fact_adolescents.htm

Wadden, T. A., Stunkard, A. J., Rich, L., Rubin, C. J., Sweidel, G., & McKinney, S. (1990). Obesity in black adolescent girls: A controlled clinical trial of treatment by diet, behavior modification, and parental support. *Pediatrics, 85*(3), 345–352.

Wang, L., Yang, Q., Lowry, R., & Weschler, H. (2003). Economic analysis of a school-based obesity prevention program. *Obesity Research, 11*, 1313–1324.

Whitaker, R. C., Wright, J. A., Pepe, M. S., Seidel, K. D., & Dietz, W. H. (1997). Predicting obesity in young adulthood from childhood and parental obesity. *New England Journal of Medicine, 337*(13), 869–873.

White, M. A., Martin, P. D., Newton, R. L., Walden, H. M., York-Crowe, E. E., Gordon, S. T., et al. (2004). Mediators of weight loss in a family-based intervention presented over the Internet. *Obesity Research, 12*(7), 1050–1059.

Williamson, D. A., Martin, P. D., White, M. A., Newton, R. L., & Walden, H. M. (2003). HIP teens: Randomized controlled trial of the efficacy of an internet-based weight management program for overweight African-American girls. *Obesity Research, 11*, A29.

Williamson, D. A., Walden, H. M., White, M. A., York-Crowe, E. E., Newton, R. L., Alfonso, A., et al. (2006). Two-year internet-based randomized controlled trial for weight loss in African-American girls. *Obesity, 14*(7), 1231–1243.

Yanovski, S. Z., & Yanovski, J. A. (2002). Obesity. *New England Journal of Medicine, 346*(8), 591–602.

Yitzhak, A., Mizrahi, S., & Avinoach, E. (2006). Laparoscopic gastric banding in adolescents. *Obesity Surgery, 16*(10), 1318–1322.

Chapter 4
Adolescent Obesity

Stephen B. Sondike

Introduction

A 14-year-old girl presents to your office for an annual physical. On reviewing the growth charts, while you notice she has always been on the higher end of the weight curve, she seems to have gained quite a bit of weight in the last year. She appears grouchy and unhappy to be at the doctor's office. On review of systems, she reports irregular periods, low back pain, and constipation. You ask the mom, also overweight if they have addressed her weight. The mother responds that she doesn't understand why her daughter is so heavy because the girl doesn't eat that much, and she wants her thyroid checked. You ask the mother to leave the room and promise confidentiality, where the girl reports she is trying to lose weight and occasionally makes herself throw up. She's also taken her friends diet pills, but nothing seems to help. She does not participate in any activities and spends most of her leisure time on the Internet talking to friends. On physical exam, her height is 50th percentile for age and her weight is well above the 95th percentile. Her calculated BMI is 38, well above the 95th percentile for age. She has a dark ring around her neck, abdominal striae, and paraspinal tenderness bilaterally. You mention these findings and how they are affected by her weight, but she just looks down at the ground. You are concerned about being too aggressive in talking about her weight because of concern of contributing to the development of an eating disorder, so you sign her school form and tell her you will see her next year.

This vignette presents a very common situation in the pediatrician's office, and medical and mental health providers are seeing this more than ever. According to the National Health and Nutrition Examination Survey (NHANES) data for the years 2003–2004, 34.3% of American adolescents aged 12–19 are at risk for overweight (>85th percentile for age BMI) or overweight (>95th percentile for age BMI). This compares unfavorably with previous data from 2001 to 2002 where only 31.1% met these criteria. This is significant when one considers that the further into childhood overweight exists, the more likely the person is to become an obese adult. Seventy-nine percent of obese 10- to 14-year-olds with at least one overweight parent will become an overweight adult. The public heath implication of the continuing supersizing of our adolescents into the future is staggering. The long-term consequences of excessive adiposity, such as atherosclerotic disease, insulin resistance, and certain cancers, are well known and described elsewhere. However, not only are overweight adolescents at risk for heath problems later in life, but

S.B. Sondike (✉)
Department of Pediatrics, West Virginia University School of Medicine, Adolescent Medicine,
Charleston Area Medical Center, Charleston, WA, USA
e-mail: ssondike@hsc.wvu.edu

L.C. James, J.C. Linton (eds.), *Handbook of Obesity Intervention for the Lifespan*,
DOI 10.1007/978-0-387-78305-5_5, © Springer Science+Business Media, LLC 2009

also immediate morbidities related to adiposity are increasing in this population, some in epidemic proportions. For example, Type 2 diabetes, previously rare in the adolescent population, has now become relatively common. This differentiates the overweight adolescent population from younger children, who most likely are healthy, regardless of their weight status.

The amount of adipocytes in the body throughout life is relatively stable. There are three stages in life where new adipocytes are added – gestation, the first year in life, and puberty. Therefore, weight gained during early life and during adolescence may have more long-term consequence than weight gained at other times. This is coupled with the fact that adolescents tend to develop idiosyncratic eating behaviors, leading to increased risk in this age group. Eating behaviors that become more common in adolescents when compared with children include the following:

- Skipping breakfast and/or lunch, then consuming food rapidly later in the day
- Eating in response to mood, that is, on being anxious, depressed, or bored
- Eating in a social context more often
- Eating more fast food
- Eating more quickly
- Discomfort with body image, leading to disordered eating, binging and restricting.

This occurs at a time when sedentary leisure time activities are becoming increasingly sophisticated. Sport-related video games are more realistic than the real thing. Social networking Internet sites such as MySpace allow kids to have active social lives without ever leaving the bedroom. Twenty-four-hour cable channels such as Nickelodeon offer programming directed toward adolescents all day, while showing advertisements for high-calorie and high-sugar foods.

Discomfort with body image is of particular concern to those treating adolescents. Studies among high-school students show that as many as half of all students at a given time are actively trying to lose weight, and as many as a quarter have actively tried unhealthy methods to lose weight, such as vomiting, laxative or diuretic use, or diet pills. This is not surprising, since ridicule of the overweight in the media persists, even though it has become a taboo to make fun of most other physical characteristics. Overweight people in the media are often presented as comic relief, usually given unpleasant personality traits such as sloppiness, clumsiness, laziness, and moral undesirability. There was even a character in a recent major movie named "Fat Bastard." Considering the toxic nature of our environment that promotes obesity, while simultaneously rejecting larger size as undesirable, it is logical that so many of our teenagers are conflicted about eating behaviors.

Association of Pubertal Changes with Obesity

It is important to remember that the adipocyte, previously believed to be a static organ used only for storage of energy, has in fact recently been shown to be an active endocrine organ. The adipocyte releases hormones such as leptin, adiponectin, and resistin, all of which have been shown to have an effect on overweight or its co-morbidities. A rapid increase in leptin release is seen in the peripubertal age ranges. This may be a factor in the increase in fat deposition around this time.

As the hormonal milieu is a major player in the development of puberty, preexisting obesity also has an effect on pubertal development. Another function of the adipocyte is the aromatization of androgens to estrogen. Because of this, adolescents who are overweight may have higher circulating estrogen levels than their lean counterparts. Overweight girls begin developing secondary sexual characteristics and menses at an earlier age than lean girls. However, overweight boys may develop secondary sexual characteristics later. Considering that early sexual development in girls is associated with more high-risk behaviors and later development in boys with low self-esteem, this is of no small concern.

Clinical Considerations

Endogenous Causes of Obesity

Although patients and parents often request a hormonal work-up for abnormal or rapid weight gain or an aggressive search for an organic cause, these are rarely found (less than 2% of the time are any organic causes found at referral to weight management programs). That being said, there are hormonal, genetic, and metabolic syndromes that are associated with excessive weight gain. In deciding who to work up, it is useful to keep the following rules in mind:

(1) Adolescents with hormonal or genetic causes for overweight are *usually short*: Almost all known hormonal or genetic syndromes associated with obesity also cause linear growth suppression.
(2) Adolescent females with irregular periods, acne, and/or excessive facial hair may have polycystic ovarian syndrome (PCOS), which will be discussed in more detail later in the chapter. PCOS is more likely the result of obesity, rather than the cause, but since it is usually treated with medications, it is mentioned here.
(3) Adolescents with obesity associated with other dysmorphic features and/or developmental delay may have a genetic syndrome.

Hormonal Causes

Hypothyroidism is the condition most people who come for weight management treatment request be ruled out. However, thyroid conditions as a cause for weight gain in overweight adolescents are extremely unusual. Suspect hypothyroidism if obesity is associated with other signs and symptoms: fatigue, depression, psychomotor retardation, or goiter. Also suspect hypothyroidism if weight gain is extremely rapid in a previously lean or normal-weight individual. In screening for hypothyroidism, a TSH is usually enough; an individual with an abnormal free thyroxine in the presence of a normal TSH is clinically euthyroid and the weight gain is likely not hormonal in origin.

Cushing's disease is the excessive release of cortisol from the adrenal glands; *Cushing's syndrome* is caused by excessive exogenous corticosteroid use (i.e., in asthma, inflammatory disease) and is associated with hypertension, abdominal striae, a round facial appearance (moon facies), and a prominent fat pad on the neck (buffalo hump). A normal 24-h urinary cortisol excretion is enough to rule out Cushing's disease.

Growth hormone deficiency (GHD) is an uncommon cause of excessive weight gain and is also associated with short stature. Insulin growth factor-1 (IGF-1) is a good screening test if GHD is suspected.

Genetic Causes

Although obesity has a strong genetic component, actual genetic disorders causing obesity are rare. Most genetic syndromes associated with overweight also cause varying degrees of developmental delay. By far, the most common of these is the *Prader–Willi Syndrome (PWS)*. PWS presents with neonatal hypotonia and is associated with obsessive behaviors and severe hyperphagia. Other physical findings include short stature, hypogonadism, and almond-shaped eyes. Other mental retardation syndromes that do not have obesity as a central component of the disorder, such as Down Syndrome and Fragile X syndrome, are associated with higher rates of obesity, as is autism. It is important to make sure adolescents with these conditions remain active and involved in activities (i.e., special olympics) and maintain a healthy home family environment.

Medications

Many medications are associated with the development of obesity. Of those commonly used in adolescents, most implicated are antipsychotics, particularly risperidol and olanzipine; injectible progesterones; oral corticosteroids; and anticonvulsants, particularly valproic acid.

Adolescent Co-morbidities

Obesity is associated with severe co-morbidities in both the short and the long term. Adolescents are unlikely to be concerned about the long-term health issues. More likely they are concerned about how they are affected in the here and now, and treatment needs to be focused on improving the immediate quality of life rather than perceived long-term benefit. Therefore, only conditions commonly seen in the adolescent will be discussed here.

Insulin resistance, metabolic syndrome, and Type 2 diabetes exist in a continuum of increasing disability of the cells to process circulating insulin, leading to increasing hypoglycemia and eventual failure of the pancreatic beta cell. A common physical manifestation of insulin resistance is *acanthosis nigricans*, a velvety hyperpigmentation found in skin folds and on the back of the neck. Often this pigmentation is mistaken for dirt by patients and parents. As mentioned, Type 2 diabetes is increasing in epidemic proportions in the adolescent populations, with an estimated 10-fold increase in incidence in the pediatric population over the last 20 years. Metabolic syndrome is the cluster of symptoms that include dyslipidemia, hypertension, and obesity, which, when existing together, increase the risk for cardiovascular disease (CVD) more than any of these increase risk individually. Up to 50% of obese adolescents may meet criteria for metabolic syndrome.

Gastrointestinal complications such as *non-alcoholic fatty liver disease* and *non-alcoholic steatorrheic hepatitis* (NASH) are diseases of fibrosis and inflammation of the hepatocyte associated with excessive adiposity and present as elevated liver function tests in children and adolescents. Up to 10% of those with NASH may progress to liver failure. *Cholelithiasis (gallstones)* are fourfold more common in the obese than in the non-obese populations. Gastroespohageal reflux disease is more common in obese adolescents than in lean ones.

Pseudotumor cerebri (benign intracranial hypertension) is a condition defined by severe headache and increased intracranial pressure with normal or small ventricles. The older in childhood it's occurrence, the higher the association with obesity. With younger children, the association is as low as 10%, but up to 90% of older teenagers with pseudotumor cerebri are obese. Treatment is by lumbar puncture.

Orthopedic problems related to obesity are common in adolescents. *Slipped capital femoral ephysisis (SCFE)* is caused by mechanical damage to the growth plate. The epiphysis of the proximal femur slips through the growth plate in a posterior direction. It presents with hip pain on external rotation of the hip. Treatment is surgical. *Blount's disease* is bowing of the tibia caused by increased weight bearing. *Flatfoot* is a collapse of the normal arch of the foot. Flatfoot is common in overweight adolescents. Low back pain is a common complaint in overweight adolescents.

Pulmonary complications include asthma and obstructive sleep apnea (OSA), a breathing disorder characterized by repeated collapse of the upper airway during sleep, with cessation of airflow at night, and daytime sleepiness due to non-restful sleep caused by the persistent nighttime awakenings. OSA is a major independent risk factor for CVD and stroke. Up to 50% of morbidly obese children may have some degree of OSA. Asthma and obesity are both increasing in the adolescent population, though the precise relationship between the two is unknown.

Reproductive complications from which obese males suffer are reproductive abnormalities including decreased sperm motility, decreased libido, and impotence. Polycystic ovarian syndrome (PCOS) occurs in obese females and is associated with, acne, hirsutism, and acanthosis nigricans. Over the long term, PCOS has been associated with infertility, CVD, Type 2 diabetes, and endometrial cancer. Even in the absence of PCOS, overweight girls often have irregular menses, likely due to the estrogenic effect of the adipocyte.

Psychological complications: The relationship between obesity and low self-esteem was previously discussed. The relationship between depression and obesity is unclear. There is certainly an association, but it is unclear whether this is a cause or an effect. Depressed people overeat, binge eat, and self-medicate with food, and being overweight causes social isolation and low self-esteem, which can lead to depression. This likely causes a vicious cycle, and it becomes difficult to address one without adequately addressing both.

Management of Adolescent Obesity

Every child presenting for a primary-care visit should have his/her height and weight measured and BMI calculated and plotted on a standard growth chart. In an overweight teen of normal height and intelligence with no dysmorphic features and on no implicated medications, a work-up for causes of excessive weight gain is not likely to be fruitful. Instead, search for co-morbidities. A fasting lipid profile and glucose, insulin, and liver function tests are good places to start. Blood pressure should be measured with a cuff of appropriate size. In girls for whom you suspect PCOS, a LH/FSH ratio of >2:1 is suggestive in the presence of a normal DHEA-S and slightly elevated free testosterone. If sleep apnea is suspected, a sleep study may be ordered.

It is important to remember with pre- and peripubertal children, weight loss is not necessarily the goal. Younger children will grow taller and grow into their weight, and around puberty there is a rapid increase in both lean body mass and fat deposition, and an expectation of weight loss may be unreasonable. Many who treat the overweight, our center included, subscribe to the concept of "health at every size (HAES)," which subscribes to the philosophy that the overall physical and psychological health is more important than a number on a scale. Data show that those who are overweight but physically fit have less morbidities than those who are lean "couch potatoes." Although population studies show differential health status with increasing BMI, this does not necessarily hold for individuals. However, HAES is not the same as size acceptance. The first word in the term is "health," and those suffering from weight-related disease should be encouraged to reduce their BMI until the condition normalizes. The treatment plan should include a combination of dietary changes, increased physical activity, and, if necessary, psychological counseling.

Dietary Treatment

For mild or moderately overweight teenagers, "diets" are usually not necessary and often counterproductive. Diets have the disadvantage of making children feel deprived, which leads to binge eating later, and stigmatization of the child, particularly when the rest of the family isn't following the diet. A better method is to encourage healthy changes for the entire family. In the vignette at the beginning of the chapter, the child's mother reported that the child didn't eat that much; however, the mother is also overweight. It is likely that this family, like many other American families, suffer from "portion distortion," which is a disturbance in the expectation of what a normal amount of food should be. It would be useful in this case to have the family complete detailed dietary histories that include weighing foods before consuming them, and educating them on standard serving sizes.

Sweetened beverages should be discouraged and juices replaced with whole fruits. Increasing fiber in the diet has been shown to aid in weight loss and lower cholesterol; changing to whole grain breads, rice, and pastas and eating five fruit and/or vegetable servings per day is a good way to achieve this goal. Snacking in front of the television leads to overeating and disturbance of cues to terminate eating; all meals and snacks should be eaten at the table. Skipping meals, particularly breakfast, is very common in teenagers and should be discouraged, as it usually leads to overeating later. Healthful eating at restaurants should be discussed. Today, even most fast food restaurants have reasonably healthy alternatives on the menu. School breakfasts and lunches are notoriously unhealthy. Encourage parents and kids to have breakfast at home, and pack a lunch for school.

Physical Activity

Physical activity in deconditioned adolescents is not necessarily "exercise." Although typical recommendations call for 30 min of aerobic exercise a day, this may be an unreasonable expectation for overweight deconditioned adolescents, who may not be physically able to comply and may become quickly discouraged. Instead, try to encourage the family to incorporate more physical activity into everyday life. For example, limit leisure time sedentary activity such as television viewing and computer activities to 2 h or less per day. Encourage walking or bicycle riding to places close enough where this is feasible. If the choice exists between stairs and elevators, take the stairs. Many larger children are uncomfortable with school physical education and request excuses. Do not provide them. This kind of physical activity can be incrementally increased until the teenager is able to take part in more formal exercise.

Cognitive Behavioral Therapy

Cognitive behavioral therapy is helpful for adolescents who have difficulty making changes on their own, those who suffer from self-esteem issues or disordered eating, and those with psychiatric co-morbidities. Motivational interviewing is an effective technique and particularly effective in adolescents who have a resistance or are precontemplative regarding making changes in lifestyle. Motivational interviewing is a style of counseling that incorporates reflexive listening and shared decision making rather than confrontation and information giving. Since so much of resistance to weight management is due to ambivalence rather than to lack of knowledge of the condition, this is an effective approach.

Treatment for Extreme Obesity

Although, in general, the concept of diet is discouraged in adolescents, in those with extreme morbid obesity or in those suffering from severe co-morbidities, strict dieting may become a necessary evil. There are several different kinds of dietary treatment programs that have been used for rapid weight loss. Also, weight loss medications and surgical approaches will be discussed.

Ketogenic diets are very low carbohydrate diets that have been studied and shown to increase the rate of weight loss in overweight adolescents. A protein sparing modified fast (PSMF) is a very low energy ketogenic diet consisting of 600–800 kcal/day with very little carbohydrate or fat. These diets are usually prescribed in an inpatient setting for 8–12 weeks and require close monitoring and the involvement of a registered dietician. Although this approach is very restrictive, there is no evidence of decreased growth velocity when instituted appropriately. Very low carbohydrate diets that do not restrict energy include the Atkins Diet and Protein Power. These diets are very popular in the lay press, but have been the subject of much controversy. In our experience, adolescents have been very successful with an Atkins-type approach, likely because they respond well to the black-and-white approach and because they do not have to count calories. Although there is a concern that the high fat content of this approach will promote increased cholesterol, clinical trials have shown that the lipid profile usually improves on an Atkins-type diet.

Low-glycemic diets are based on altering the quality rather than the quantity of carbohydrates in the diet. The glycemic index (GI) is an experimentally derived measure of the insulin response to a certain food. In general, the more processed a carbohydrate source in a food, the higher the GI. For example, whole grains have a lower GI than white flour, and steel-cut oats a lower GI than instant oatmeal. The GI approach is also controversial, because critics suggest that since individual foods are measured, the effect when foods are mixed together in a regular diet is uncertain. However, controlled clinical trials in children and adolescents have shown increased weight loss in low GI diets when compared with low-fat diets. Again, in adolescents, this approach, by focusing on the type rather than quantity of foods, has the advantage of not requiring calorie counting, which makes teens feel restricted. Also, a low GI diet, in contrast with the Atkins diet, encourages fruit and vegetable intake and discourages saturated fat intake, which makes this approach more sustainable in the long term.

Medications

Two medications are approved for weight loss in adolescents: orlistat (Xenical) and sibutramine (Meridia). Orlistat, a fat absorption blocker, is available in both prescription and over-the-counter preparations. Side effects are usually related to malabsorption of fats and include steatorrhea, bloating, flatulence, and fat-soluable vitamin malnutrition and are increased with higher fat intake. Although in some adolescents, the negative conditioning associated with uncomfortable side effects from eating fatty foods is a benefit, often adolescents discontinue orlistat due to discomfort rather than decrease fat intake. Sibutamine is a norephinephrine and serotonin uptake inhibitor that works centrally to decrease appetite. Side effects include increased pulse rate and blood pressure, insomnia, anxiety, and sleep disturbance. Sibutramine cannot be used in conjunction with serotonin reuptake inhibitors or MAO inhibitors. Sibutramine is approved for ages 16 and higher. Several medications that have not been approved for weight loss but have some weight loss properties have been used off-label for weight control. These include metformin (Glucophage), an insulin sensitizer; topirimate (Topamax), an anticonvulsant; and fluoxitine (Prozac), an antidepressant. If a medication from one of these classes is indicated in an overweight adolescent, it might be of benefit to choose one of these. Teenagers commonly turn to herbal dietary supplements that promise to help them lose weight. Usually, these are some combination of caffeine, herbal psychostimulants (such as guarana), and/or fiber. These are usually expensive and unlikely to be of benefit. Be especially cautious of supplements containing ephedrine or ma huang. Although removed from the market in the United States, these preparations are readily available on the black market or over the Internet. Use of these preparations has been associated with hypertension, arrhythmias, stroke, and sudden death. Chromium is a supplement long believed to possess weight loss properties, but scientific studies so far have shown no benefit.

In general, we do not recommend weight loss medications and supplements for our adolescent populations. First, many adolescents requesting a "diet pill" are not fully committed to lifestyle changes; the effects of medications are subtle and are unlikely to be effective in this context. Second, long-term benefits for adolescents have not conclusively been shown. In both these cases, it is uncertain that the benefits would outweigh the risks. If we do prescribe medications, it is usually only after a teen and family has shown commitment to lifestyle changes first.

Bariatric Surgery

Bariatric surgery is a controversial option in adolescents, but can be considered as a last resort for those who have morbid obesity with life-threatening complications. A recent expert panel recommendation suggested that surgery only be considered in an adolescent if he/she has reached skeletal maturity, has a BMI over 50, has at least 6 months of compliance in a weight management program, and has a supportive family environment. The Roux-Y gastroplasty is the recommended procedure because it has the most effective rate of weight loss, although this procedure is also associated with higher rates of morbidity and side effects. Adjustable gastric banding (often called "lap-band") has lower morbidity rates but slower weight loss. This procedure is currently under study for adolescents.

Summary

Obesity is a major issue in the adolescent population and is related to significant morbidities in both the immediate and the long term. Poor self-esteem and development of disordered eating behaviors are of particular concern. Healthy eating behaviors and daily physical activity are the usually recommended treatments, although for some, stricter dieting or medications may be required. Bariatric surgery is usually withheld except for the most extreme, life-threatening cases. Cognitive behavioral therapy and motivational interviewing are useful adjuncts in treatment, particularly for those ambivalent about making necessary changes.

Chapter 5
Innovations in Preventing and Treating Obesity in Children and Adolescents: The Role of Physical Activity Interventions

Dawn K. Wilson and Duncan C. Meyers

Introduction

Over the past two decades, the prevalence of overweight and obesity have increased dramatically in US youth (Freedman, Khan, Serdula, Oden, & Dietz, 2006; Ogden et al., 2006). In 2003–2004, 17.1% of US children and adolescents were overweight or obese with an increase in prevalence rate of 13.8% in females and 14.0% in males from 1999 to 2004 (Ogden et al., 2006). It has also been suggested that this increasing rate of obesity has also been associated with an increasing prevalence of type 2 diabetes mellitus, high blood pressure, high cholesterol, and certain cancers (Cook, Weitzman, Auinger, Nguyen, & Dietz, 2003; Hanevold, Waller, Daniels, Portman, & Sorof, 2005; Must & Strauss, 1999; Wabitsch, 2000). Thus, obesity prevention and intervention programs are needed to decrease this increasing rate of obesity in youth.

Physical inactivity and unhealthy diet have been shown to be linked to serious public health problems such as obesity, chronic disease, morbidity, and mortality. National studies have shown that engaging in healthy diet and physically active lifestyles can significantly reduce the risks of chronic disease, morbidity, and mortality. For example, moderate-intensity physical activity (PA) that is consistently incorporated into routine activities of daily living can improve fitness and prevent leading causes of death and disability, including obesity (Center for Disease Control and Prevention, 2000; Pate et al., 1995). Regular PA reduces the risk for cardiovascular morbidity and all-cause mortality and helps to maintain and enhance weight loss (US DHHS, 2000). Prospective studies indicate that regular PA reduces the risk of non-insulin-dependent diabetes mellitus and improves insulin sensitivity (Manson et al., 1992, 1991).

Previous investigators have focused on studying how insufficient energy expenditure relative to energy intake and inappropriate consumption of selected nutrients or foods (e.g., excess calories, dietary fat) are related to obesity. National studies have shown that specific contributions of dietary factors to the onset of obesity are unclear. Several studies have showed no relationship between changes in dietary intake and increases in obesity (Nicklas et al., 2004a, 2004b). Other investigators have also reported that despite increasing body weight, total reported energy intake was unchanged (Nicklas, Elkasabany, Srinivasan, & Berenson, 2001) although reported consumption of energy-dense snacks increased in youth (Jahns, Siega-Riz, & Popkin, 2001; Nicklas et al., 2001). Although some investigators have reported that fast food consumption has been associated with higher energy intake, higher

D.K. Wilson (✉)
Department of Psychology, Barnwell College, University of South Carolina, Columbia, SC 29208, USA
e-mail: wilsondk@mailbox.sc.edu

L.C. James, J.C. Linton (eds.), *Handbook of Obesity Intervention for the Lifespan*,
DOI 10.1007/978-0-387-78305-5_6, © Springer Science+Business Media, LLC 2009

intake of soft drinks, and lower intake of fruit, vegetables, grains, and milk, no connection has been directly linked to the increasing rate of obesity in youth (French, Story, Neumark-Sztainer, Fulkerson, & Hannan, 2001).

Physical inactivity has also been proposed to be a component of total energy expenditure and an important factor to consider in understanding obesity. In a review by Taylor and Sallis (1997), it was reported that only 50% of youth were meeting the national guidelines of engaging in vigorous PA for 3 or more days per week for at least 20 min/day. In addition, previous studies indicate that 43% of adolescents report viewing television more than 2 h/day, making television viewing a major contributor to a sedentary lifestyle (US DHHS, 1999). In addition, as youth approach adolescence, PA rates decline (Kimm et al., 2000).

There have been a relatively large number of studies examining the prevalence of PA in children and adolescents. The literature on behavioral PA interventions, however, has demonstrated inconsistent effects on increasing PA in children and adolescents. In general, intervention studies have demonstrated only modest changes in youth's PA during physical education (PE) class time but little change in overall PA outside of school class time. The purpose of this chapter is to review obesity prevention and treatment studies in children and adolescents and highlight the innovative role of PA interventions that may be useful to clinicians.

Importance of Physical Activity in Obesity Prevention and Intervention Studies

Recent literature reviews of efforts to prevent and treat obesity and overweight in child and adolescent populations suggest that engagement in PA is critical (American Dietetic Association, 2006; Flynn et al., 2006). These reviews strongly suggest apparent benefits of providing multi-component interventions that include PA for families when children are young (5–12 years old) and benefits of providing school-based multi-component interventions including PA for youth in high school. Schools have been found to be critical setting for prevention and intervention programming where health status indicators – such as BMI and chronic disease risk factors – can be positively impacted. Beyond schools, there are surprisingly large gaps in the literature for interventions in home and community settings, limiting the understanding of the effectiveness of interventions in such environments. Additional gaps in the literature surround children 0–6 years of age, males, and minorities, and less is known regarding effective obesity prevention and interventions for these population subgroups. In an effort to lessen one of these gaps, Bluford, Sherry, and Scanlon (2007) reviewed interventions to change weight status or body fat for children aged 2–6 years. These authors found that the heterogeneity of frameworks/theories, strategies, and outcome measures used in studies made it difficult to identify any single effective strategy as compared to others. While their review was inconclusive, the importance of parent involvement for younger children was apparent.

Reviews specific to prevention of obesity and overweight in children and adolescents also strongly suggest inclusion of PA within a multi-component strategy. Identifying effective strategies is an important pursuit, given that a meta-analysis of obesity prevention programs (Stice, Shaw, & Marti, 2006) found that 79% of the programs they evaluated did not produce statistically reliable weight gain prevention effects. The authors state that it is imperative to focus on the 21% of the prevention programs that produced significant weight gain prevention effects, and additional reviews have been conducted to help identify what might be the aspects of successful childhood overweight prevention programs (e.g., Budd & Volpe, 2006; Doak, Visscher, Renders, & Seidell, 2006). Findings for reviews of successful childhood overweight prevention programs state that – for older students – classroom instruction and PE can promote moderate-to-vigorous PA, especially for teenage girls. For younger children, the largest effects included a parental involvement component, and there seems to be a benefit from behavior change programs that reduce sedentary behavior. Although evidence suggests that eating behaviors are shaped by caregivers, few broad-based interventions target parents or home environments. These reviews suggest that family-based interventions combining education with behavior modification are most successful and propose that best practice for obesity prevention is an intervention that includes both PA and diet.

Obesity Prevention Studies with Physical Activity Components

Given the importance attributed to PA in the prevention literature, understanding factors that increase it are essential to improving outcomes. Reviews of efforts to promoting PA (e.g., Salmon, Booth, Phongsavan, Murphy, & Timperio, 2007; van Sluijs, McMinn, & Griffin, 2008) suggest that – for children – studies that included increased PA in PE classes and incorporated curriculum and/or environmental changes were more effective than curriculum-only programs. Some evidence of effect was shown for environmental interventions and those targeted at children from low socioeconomic backgrounds. Among adolescents, published evidence to date suggests that a multilevel approach to promoting PA – combining school-based interventions with family and community involvement and educational interventions with policy and environmental changes – is likely to be effective and should be promoted. It has also been suggested that interventions in primary-care settings, tailored advice, or brief counseling appear to be most effective. Interventions in the family setting showed weak positive trends, and this may be due to the large percentage of these studies that were pilot studies and were not adequately powered.

Table 5.1 presents a summary of key obesity prevention studies that highlights the age group, study sample, intervention components, outcomes, and recommendations for clinical practice. In particular the studies were selected for inclusion in this table because they represent programs that have demonstrated modest-to-strong effectiveness across youth in preschool, elementary-school, middle-school, and high-school. Highlighted in the table are the innovative elements related to the PA component of each obesity prevention program. Recommendations are highlighted from each study to assist clinicians and health-care providers in developing effective obesity prevention programs for youth. In general, the studies in Table 5.1 show the importance of including parents, integrating multi-component approaches, and incorporating PA in creative and fun ways when developing obesity prevention programs for youth of all ages.

Obesity Intervention Studies with Physical Activity Components

Reviews of empirical literature related to pediatric obesity and overweight intervention also suggest that multi-component interventions include a PA component. For example, Jelalian, Wember, Bungeroth, and Birmaher (2007) found that comprehensive behavioral interventions that include dietary prescription, PA, and/or decreased sedentary behavior and behavior modification targeted at both children and parents or parents alone can be

Table 5.1 Summary of obesity prevention studies with physical activity components

Author	Age group (years)	Sample	Components of intervention	Primary outcomes	Findings	Recommendations
Fitzgibbon et al. (2005) (Hip-Hop to Health Jr.)	Preschool (ages 3–5 years)	300 children (African American) from low-income families enrolled in one of 12 Head Start Programs	RCT: (1) weight control intervention (WCI) 14-week program: healthy eating, PA (Hip Hop dance) parent newsletter or (2) general health intervention (GHI)	BMI, PA (assessed by parents), dietary intake (parental report taken by dietitian)	No effects at post-intervention At 1 year post-intervention, increase in mean adjusted BMI was significantly different for WCI vs. GHI (0.06 kg/m^2 vs. 0.59 kg/m^2) At 2 year post-intervention, the mean increase in BMI was 0.54 kg/m^2 higher ($p < 0.05$) for the GHI group as compared to the WCI group.	This approach highlights the importance of culturally based PA programs such as Hip Hop for African-American youth in preventing increases in BMI. The lack of differences between WCI and GHI for any of the dietary measures or PA measures could be due to use of a single dietary recall and a non-validated PA measure. These results were not replicated in Head Start Programs comprised of predominantly Latino preschoolers.
Sääkslahti et al. (2004) (SPAN)	Preschool (age 4 years)	228 children	Not RCT: (1) intervention ($n =$ 116; 48% boys) 1-h meetings with the parents, delivery of print materials, PA demonstration with children, and a unique radio	PA diary	The use of a physical activity diary indicated that children in the intervention group spent more time playing outdoors ($p = 0.041$) than children in the	Difficult to say whether these findings can be generalized, but involving parents proved to be important in increasing outdoor play in children.

Table 5.1 (continued)

Author	Age group (years)	Sample	Components of intervention	Primary outcomes	Findings	Recommendations
			program with the parents (2) control (*n* = 112; 55% boys) no intervention		control group (3.11 vs. 1.99 h/weekend)	
Manios, Moschandreas, Hatzis, and Kafatos (2002) (based on Know Your Body)	School age (ages 5–6 years)	831 children enrolled in 1 of 40 schools in Crete, Greece	Not RCT: (1) schools assigned as the intervention group (IG) curriculum based on Know Your Body program, two PA lessons/week, classroom sessions, homework activities with parents, and parental meetings (2) Control group (CG) no program	*At 6-year follow-up:* BMI, skin fold (triceps, biceps, suprailiac), self-report PA, fitness indices, daily nutrient intakes, serum lipids	Significantly greater increase in time spent in MVPA for IG vs. CG (adjusted mean increases of 281.3 vs. 174.5 min/week) Significantly greater improvements in weight, height, BMI, and skin folds for IG vs. CG	A successful long-term intervention that involved school curriculum, structured PA within school, homework with parents, and face-to-face meetings with parents. Speaks to the potential long-term effects that may result from multi-component prevention efforts.
Taylor et al. (2007) (APPLE Project)	School age (ages 5–12 years)	730 New Zealand children (82% White) attending 1 of 7 schools	Not RCT (1) Four intervention schools – nutrition education and PA program that focused on non-curricula- lifestyle-based activities facilitated by activity coordinators (2) Three control schools that	Assessed at baseline, 1- and 2-year follow-up: BMI, waist circumference, blood pressure, diet, PA	BMI *z* score was significantly lower in intervention children than in control children by a mean of 0.09 kg/m^2 (95% CI: 0.01, 0.18) after 1 year and 0.26 kg/m^2 (95% CI: 0.21, 0.32) at 2 years A significant interaction was shown between intervention group	A relatively simple approach, providing activity coordinators and basic nutrition education in schools, can significantly reduce the rate of excessive weight gain in children, although this may be limited to those not initially overweight.

Table 5.1 (continued)

Author	Age group (years)	Sample	Components of intervention	Primary outcomes	Findings	Recommendations
		received funds for school equipment			and overweight status; mean **BMI** z score was reduced in normal-weight (-0.29; 95% CI: -0.38, -0.21) but not overweight (-0.02; 95%CI: -0.16, 0.12).	
Harrell et al. (1996)	School age (ages 8–9 years)	1,274 3rd and 4th graders (48% boys) attending 1 of 12 schools in both rural and urban areas	RCT: schools stratified by region were assigned to either: (1) 8-week intervention consisting of interactive interventions consisting of mandated increases in PA intervention three times per week and psychoeducation delivered twice per week. (2) Control condition receiving usual health instruction	BMI, cholesterol, BP, TSF, subscapular skin fold, PA, knowledge	No effects for BMI compared to control group receiving regular health education curriculum Skin fold (transformed via natural log) of triceps and subscapular were significantly different between intervention and control	The strong focus on PA in this study may have impacted skin fold parameters more so the BMI per se.
Luepker et al. (1996) (CATCH)	School age (ages 8–10 years)	3,959 3rd through 5th graders enrolled in 1 of 96 schools	RCT: (1) 56 intervention and 40 control elementary schools. 28 intervention	BMI, blood pressure, cholesterol, diet, PA, knowledge, self-efficacy, social support, and changes in school	No significant effects for BMI compared to matched control group Participants in the intervention schools	While the intervention is effective for promoting PA during PE, it is unclear whether it is also effective in

Table 5.1 (continued)

Author	Age group (years)	Sample	Components of intervention	Primary outcomes	Findings	Recommendations
			schools mandated PA increases during PE classes, health promotion curriculum, and food service changes. (2) Other half of the intervention schools ($n = 28$) same program with a family-based education component.	lunch and PE programs	were observed to engage in PA of increased intensity in PE compared to control schools ($p <$ 0.05). At post-assessment intervention students reported significantly more daily vigorous activity than controls (58.6 min vs. 46.5 min; $p <$ 0.01).	promoting children's overall PA No significant effects for BMI compared to matched control group Nice example of multi-component program
Prochaska and Sallis (2004)	School age ($M =$ 12.2 years; $SD =$ 0.9)	138 children in 6–8th grades (65% female)	RCT: Participants randomly assigned within classrooms to: (1) single-behavior PA intervention ($n =$ 46) based on computer-aided health education sessions, tailored feedback with individual behavior plans plus nutrition (2) Multiple-behavior PA and nutrition (PAN; $n = 46$) same as above plus a nutrition	Outcomes assessed baseline to 3-month follow-up Change in PA accelerometer data 3-day dietary recording baseline to 3-month follow-up	The PAN and PA interventions were efficacious in increasing boys' ($p <$ 0.001) but not girls' PA relative to the control condition	Suggests that computer-based, tailored feedback, and a brief one-time 30 min intervention is effective in boys.

Table 5.1 (continued)

Author	Age group (years)	Sample	Components of intervention	Primary outcomes	Findings	Recommendations
			intervention (3) No treatment control ($n = 46$)			
Gortmaker et al. (1999) (Planet Health)	School age (age 11–12 years)	1,295 children (48% female; 66% white) enrolled in 1 of 10 schools	RCT: schools were matched and then randomized to receive 2 years of either: (1) intervention consisting of classroom lessons, television viewing reduction campaign, PA-related activities delivered in PE classes or (2) control condition receiving usual health curricula and PE classes.	% obesity, BMI, triceps skin fold (TSF), subscapular skin folds, PA, television viewing, dietary intake	Over the 2-school-year intervention periods, obesity prevalence among female students in the intervention schools declined from 23.6% to 20.3% while control schools increased from 21.5% to 23.7%. Data indicated significantly greater remission for female students who were obese in intervention vs. control schools.	Reduction in obesity for girls, but not boys Over the 21-month period, only 33 incident cases of obesity occurred (13 among intervention girls). Significant differences in remission of obesity between intervention and control in females was still detected Strong support for the importance of reducing television watching as well as increasing PA.
Sallis et al. (2003) (M-SPAN)	School age (age 11–13 years)	6th–8th grade students from 24 RCT: schools (mean 1109 per school)	(1) 12 intervention schools received a 2-year environmental and policy intervention focusing on increasing PA in PE classes and during leisure time (increased	Observed PA (SOPLAY and SOFIT), parent and student reported PA, school menu documentation, recipes and package labels of school lunches	Gender-specific analyses revealed the time by condition interaction was significant for boys ($p < 0.01$), and intervention schools were observed to engage in MVPA	Shows the relevance of PA interventions for boys (relative to girls), but little impact on BMI.

Table 5.1 (continued)

Author	Age group (years)	Sample	Components of intervention	Primary outcomes	Findings	Recommendations
			supervision, equipment, and activities), and reducing saturated dietary fat purchased at or brought to school; (2) 12 control schools received usual curriculum		more so than those in control schools ($d = 1.10$).	
Pate et al. (2005) (LEAP)	Adolescent ($M = 13.6$ years; $SD = 0.6$)	2,744 9th Grade girls attending 1 of 22 schools (48.7% African American, 46.7% White)	RCT: Schools paired and randomized to: (1) 1-year multi-component intervention: instructional practices and the school environment to increase support for PA among girls school-wide (2) Regular PE classes	PA (3DPAR), BMI	After adjusting for baseline values and other covariates, girls in the LEAP intervention schools participated in a significantly higher average of 1 or more 30-min blocks of vigorous physical activity per day during the 3-day recall period compared to girls in the control schools ($p < 0.05$)	First to show that a school-based intervention can increase regular participation in vigorous PA among high-school girls. Demonstrates that school programs can promote PA among adolescent girls

RCT: randomized clinical trial; PA: physical activity; M = mean; SD = standard deviation; d = Cohen's d (effectsize) effective treatments for pediatric obesity. For children, a major limitation of obesity treatment literature is the limited number of intervention studies with control groups that focus on weight loss (Snethen, Broome, & Cashin, 2006). There is also a lack of maintenance programs to provide ongoing treatment and support to children after they have reached their goals. For treatment of adolescent obesity, there is insufficient evidence to conclude that any one treatment approach or a combination of approaches is superior in the management of adolescent obesity (Tsiros, Sinn, Coates, Howe, & Buckley, 2008). Studies in this area have provided conflicting results, in some instances suggesting that adolescents may be more responsive without parents present (e.g., Brownell, Kelman, & Stunkard, 1983), whereas other studies have concluded that the level of parental involvement had no effect on treatment outcomes (Wadden et al., 1990). Despite inconclusive findings, the use of psychological intervention such as behavior therapy and cognitive behavioral therapy combined with strategies to improve diet and PA show promise, particularly in their potential for long-term maintenance of behaviors that assist in maintaining a healthy weight (Tsiros et al., 2008).

Reviews of obesity and overweight prevention and treatment literature consistently highlight the importance of PA. The effectiveness of PA as an efficacious strategy for weight management and reduction of body composition variables in children and adolescents is strengthened by additional meta-analyses recently conducted (Atlantis, Barnes, & Singh, 2006; LeMura & Maziekas, 2002). While it is suggested that PA has a modest-to-strong impact on percentage body fat, body mass, decreased BMI, and increased fat-free mass in obese children, it should be noted that these meta-analyses are limited by the small number of randomized trials currently available. These studies are also limited by inconsistent reporting of sample characteristics for studies in the literature. The studies analyzed by LeMura and Maziekas (2002) indicated that the most favorable alterations in body composition occur with low-intensity, longer duration aerobic exercise combined with high-repetition resistance training. Conversely, Atlantis and colleagues (2006) found that an aerobic prescription of 155–180 min/week of moderate-to-high-intensity PA seems most effective for reducing body fat in overweight children and adolescents aged 8–15 years. Despite the different messages sent regarding the intensity of PA that may be most efficacious, these analyses highlight the benefit of prescribing PA as part of a strategy to reduce adiposity, especially in conjunction with behavioral strategies (e.g., support from family, dietary classes, reduction of sedentary behaviors).

Table 5.2 presents a summary of key obesity treatment studies that highlights the age group, study sample, intervention components, outcomes, and recommendations for clinical practice. In particular the studies were selected for inclusion in this table because they represent programs that have demonstrated modest-to-strong effectiveness across youth of preschool, elementary school, middle-school, and high-school age. Highlighted in the table are the innovative elements related to the PA component of each obesity prevention program. Recommendations are highlighted from each study to assist clinicians and health-care providers in developing effective obesity prevention programs for youth.

In general, there is strong evidence to recommend multi-component obesity interventions for children and adolescents, which include parent training, dietary/nutritional education, PA in conjunction with methods to reduce sedentary behaviors, and behavior counseling (self-monitoring, goal setting, "Stop Light" diet). Most studies used a combination of dietary counseling, PA, and behavioral interventions (self-monitoring, modeling, goal setting, contingency management). Despite evidence for effectiveness of obesity

Table 5.2 Summary of obesity interventions with a physical activity component

Author	Age group	Sample	Components of intervention	Primary outcomes	Findings	Recommendations
Epstein, Wing, Koeske, Andrasik, and Ossip (1981) (follow-up Epstein, Valoski, Wing, & McCurley, 1994)	School age (6–12 years)	Child (n = 56) and parents (n = 46) who were 15–80% overweight at baseline	RCT: Participants assigned to (1) parent/child targeted for contingency management for behavior and weight change (n = 30), (2) child-only target (n = 26), or (3) non-specific target (n = 30). Each group participated in a 14-session treatment program over 6 months. Subjects in each group were given information on aerobic exercise, and diet.	Percentage overweight	At both 5- and 10-year follow-ups, parent-and-child group had significantly greater decreases in the percentage overweight than the non-specific control Percentages of children in the parent-and-child, child-only, and control groups that maintained decreases of less than 20% overweight were 43%, 22%, and 29%, respectively.	Evidence suggests that treatments targeting and reinforcing change in habits and weight loss in obese parents and children together are superior over 10 years to treatments that focus solely on the child's habits and weight change. These results were demonstrated independent of parental success, as well as to a control treatment that targets and reinforces the family members for attendance only.
Golan, Weizman, Apter, and Fainaru, (1998) (follow-up Golan & Crow, 2004)	School age (6–11 years)	60 Israeli children (62% female) and their parents; children > 20% of the recommended weight-for-age, weight-for-height	RCT: Children matched for sex and age were randomly assigned to (1) Parent-only group (only parents were targeted) participating in 14 diet PA educational group sessions; or (2) Child-only	Percentage overweight, weight loss, body frame, family completed 7-day food diaries, social demographic questionnaire, family eating and activity habits questionnaire	Children in the parent-only group achieved a significantly higher reduction in percent overweight compared with the children in the child-only group (14.6% vs. 8.43%; p < 0.05) 7 years after program termination	Shows importance of focusing parents on skill training and role modeling appropriate behaviors.

Table 5.2 (continued)

Author	Age group	Sample	Components of intervention	Primary outcomes	Findings	Recommendations
			group (children were targeted) prescribed a diet providing 1500 kcal/d participating in thirty group diet and PA sessions were led by a clinical dietitian.		(participants were 14–19 years old) both treatment conditions demonstrated substantial weight loss.	
Epstein, Wing, Koeske, and Valoski (1984) (follow-up Epstein, Valoski, Wing, & McCurley, 1994)	School age (8–12 years)	Child and parents from 53 families who were 15–80% overweight at baseline	RCT: Children were randomized to (1) Traffic light diet (Diet) (2) Diet combined with lifestyle-change exercise (Diet + Exercise) program. Each group participated in a 15-session treatment program, distributed over 20 weeks with biweekly meetings. These interventions were compared to wait-list controls	BMI	Diet along and Diet + Exercise superior percentage overweight change to wait-list control in 10-year follow-up (p^2.05)	Results suggest preliminary evidence that exercise enhances the long-term effects of diet interventions for obese children. This approach may not generalize to minority populations.
Nemet et al., (2005)	School age/ adolescent (6–16 years)	40 Israeli children and adolescents	RCT: age and gender matched participants assigned to (1) combined dietary-behavioral-physical	Nutritional assessment, Habitual activity assessment, Fitness	Significant difference between intervention and control for: Body weight (0.6 ± 6.0 kg vs. 5.3 ± 2.7 kg) BMI (−1.7 ±	First study to show promise of increasing leisure time PA.

Table 5.2 (continued)

Author	Age group	Sample	Components of intervention	Primary outcomes	Findings	Recommendations
			activity intervention (Intervention) (2) Control ($n = 20$) referrec to an ambulatory nutritional consultation	assessment, Serum lipid levels	2.3 kg/m^2 vs. 0.6 ± 0.9 kg/m^2) Significant increase in leisure-time PA among the intervention participants compared to controls	
Savoye et al. (2007) Bright Bodies	School age/children & adolescent (8–16 years)	135 participants (34% Caucasian, 36% African American, 29% Hispanic, 58% Female) BMI >95th percentile for age and sex	RCT: (1) Weight management group (WM; $n = 105$) 6 month bi-weekly intensive family-based program including exercise, nutrition, and behavior modification along with brief psychosocial counseling by a social worker. (2) Control ($n = 69$) which received traditional clinical weight management counseling every 6 months	Change in weight, BMI, body fat, insulin resistance (HOMA-IR)	WM demonstrated increases in the following compared to control: Mean weight (+0.3 kg [−1.4 to 2.0] vs. + 7.7 kg [5.3 to 10.0], $p < 0.001$) BMI (−1.7 [−2.3 to−1.1] vs. + 1.6 [0.8 to 2.3], $p < 0.001$) Body fat (−3.7 kg [−5.4 to−2.1] vs. +5.5 kg [3.2 to 7.8], $p < 0.001$) HOMA-IR (−1.52 [−1.93 to−1.01] vs. +0.90 [−0.07 to 2.05], $p < 0.001$)	Intervention group experienced no weight gain over 12 months, a 4% (3.7 kg) reduction in body fat and a modest fall in BMI. Shows impact of weight loss on insulin resistance.

Table 5.2 (continued)

Author	Age group	Sample	Components of intervention	Primary outcomes	Findings	Recommendations
Saelens et al. (2002)	School age/ adolescent (12 to 16 years)	44 overweight adolescents (41% female, 71% White, 16% Hispanic, 4.5% African American) > 89th percentile BMI for age and sex	RCT: (1) Health Habits (HH) learning self-monitoring assisted with computer and telephone format, behavioral skills manual, and materials sent to parents; (2) Typical Care (TC) which received pediatrician recommendations for healthful eating and PA	Dietary intake, PA, 7-day PAR interview, sedentary behaviors, problematic eating	Group by time interaction from baseline to post-treatment for BMI ($p < 0.05$; effect size $f = 0.40$), and scores significantly increased among TC adolescents compared with the slight decrease of BMI z scores among HH adolescents.	First study to integrate clinicians into the study treatment design. Further work is need in this area.

RCT: randomized clinical trial; PA: physical activity; HOMA-IR = Homeostasis Model Assessment of Insulin Resistance.

interventions, there is a lack of support for long-term weight loss as a result of these efforts. It may be that it is reasonable to expect a greater impact over a shorter period of time on weight status/adiposity among self-selecting highly motivated groups than among a population sample, regardless of the nature of the intervention (American Dietetic Association, 2006).

Summary and Conclusions

There are several interesting themes that are worth commenting on in terms of potential future directions for the field. First, in general, the prevention and intervention studies reviewed in this chapter demonstrated the important role of better understanding the integration of environmental and social resources in multi-component PA and dietary interventions. Thus, these studies suggest that investigators and clinicians consider broader conceptual issues in the context of developing obesity prevention and intervention programs beyond solely focusing on interpersonal factors such as intentions, motivation, and self-efficacy constructs. This chapter sets the stage for future investigators to study how biological, social, and environmental context of ones' world impact or interact with their interpersonal beliefs in changing long-term behavior.

There are a number of limitations with previous studies that should be mentioned. Low power due to having a small number of participants is among many frequent methodological flaws seen in interventions in children and adolescents. In addition, other limitations include infrequent inclusion of baseline data, poor study design (e.g., no control group or baseline data), atheorctical intervention programs, and use of PA measures of unknown reliability or validity (Salmon et al., 2007). Additional limitations of PA intervention research include lack of follow-up analyses, lack of investigations of differential effects for population subgroups (e.g., based on sex or ethnicity), and failure to account for clustering due to randomization at the school level with appropriate statistical analyses (Thomas, 2006). In light of these limitations, the literature suggests that a promising preventive strategy for increasing PA may be creating lifestyle patterns of physical fitness in childhood youth that will extend into adulthood.

A recurrent theme in the studies reviewed in this chapter is the importance of PA as a strategy to prevent and treat obesity in children and adolescents. The current review adds to previous literature as it focuses specifically on the contribution of PA in developing effective obesity prevention and treatment programs for youth. Much of the evidence with respect to effectiveness of PA interventions among youth is still emerging. The current review was purposely inclusive of less rigorous designs in the interest of communicating the range of strategies that have been included in trials. Incorporating innovative PA components into obesity prevention and treatment interventions shows promise for engaging youth in positive lifestyle changes that may reduce their risk of developing obesity.

Acknowledgment This article was support by a grant (R01 HD 045693) funded by the National Institutes of Child Health and Human Development to Dawn K. Wilson, Ph.D. Send reprint requests to Dawn K. Wilson, Ph.D., professor, Department of Psychology, Barnwell College, University of South Carolina, Columbia, SC 29208; email address: wilsondk@mailbox.sc.edu.

References

American Dietetic Association. (2006). Position of the American Dietetic Association: Individual-, family-, school-, and community-based interventions for pediatric overweight. *Journal of the American Dietetic Association, 106*, 925–945.

Atlantis, E., Barnes, E. H., & Singh, M. A. (2006) Efficacy of exercise for treating overweight in children and adolescents: A systematic review. *International Journal of Obesity, 30*, 1027–1040.

Bluford, D. A. A., Sherry, B., & Scanlon, K. S. (2007). Interventions to prevent or treat obesity in preschool children: A review of evaluated programs. *Obesity, 15*, 1356–1372.

Brownell, K. D., Kelman, J. H., & Stunkard, A. J. (1983). Treatment of obese children with and without their mothers: Changes in weight and blood pressure. *Pediatrics, 71*, 515–523.

Budd, G. M., & Volpe, S. L. (2006). School-based obesity prevention: Research, challenges, and recommendations. *Journal of School Health, 76*, 485–495.

Center for Disease Control and Prevention. (2000). *Physical activity and good nutrition: Essential elements for good health.* Atlanta, BA. Retrieved from: http://www.cdc.gov/nccdphp/dnpa/dnpaaag:htm

Cook, S., Weitzman, M., Auinger, P., Nguyen, M., & Deitz, W. H. (2003). Prevalence of a metabolic syndrome phenotype in adolescents: findings from the Third National Health and Nutrition Examination Survey, 1988–1994. *Archives of Pediatric Medicine, 157*, 821–827.

Doak, C. M., Visscher, T. L. S., Renders, C. M., & Seidell, J. C. (2006). The prevention of overweight and obesity in children and adolescents: A review of interventions and programmes. *Obesity Reviews, 7*, 111–136.

Epstein, L. H., Valoski, A., Wing, R. R., & McCurley, J. (1994). Ten-year outcomes of behavioral family-based treatment for childhood obesity. *Health Psychology, 13*, 373–383.

Epstein, L. H., Wing, R. R., Koeske, R., Andrasik, F., & Ossip, D. J. (1981). Child and parent weight loss in family-based behavioral modification programs. *Journal of Consulting and Clinical Psychology, 49*, 674–685.

Epstein, L. H., Wing, R. R., Koeske, R., & Valoski, A. (1984). The effects of diet plus exercise on weight change in parents and children. *Journal of Consulting and Clinical Psychology, 52*, 429–437.

Fitzgibbon, M., Stolley, M., Schiffer, L., Van Horn, L., Kauf erChristoffel, K., & Dyer, A. (2005). Two-year follow-up results for Hip-Hop to Health Jr.: A randomized controlled trial for overweight prevention in preschool minority children. *Journal of Pediatrics, 146*, 618–625.

Flynn, M. A. T., McNeil, D. A., Maloff, B., Mutasingwa, D., Wu, M., Ford, C., et al. (2006). Reducing obesity and related chronic disease risk in children and youth: A synthesis of evidence with 'best practice' recommendations. *Obesity Reviews, 7*(Supp. 1), 7–66

Freedman, D. S., Khan, L. K., Serdula, J. K., Ogden, C. L., & Dietz, W. H. (2006). Racial and ethnic differences in secular trends for childhood BMI, weight, and height. *Obesity, 14*(2), 301–308.

French, S. A., Story, M., Neumark-Sztainer, D., Fulkerson, J. A., & Hannan, P., (2001). Fast food restaurant use among adolescents: associations with nutrient intake, food choices and behavioral and psychosocial variables. *International Journal of Obesity and Related Metabolic Disorders,25*(12), 1823–1833.

Golan, M., & Crow, S. (2004). Targeting parents exclusively in the treatment of childhood obesity: Long-term results. *Obesity Research, 12*, 357–361.

Golan, M., Weizman, A., Apter A., & Fainaru, M. (1998). Parents as the exclusive agents of change in the treatment of childhood obesity. *American Journal of Clinical Nutrition, 67*, 1130–1135.

Gortmaker, S. L., Peterson, K., Wiecha, J., Sobol, A. M., Dixit, S., Fox, M. K.,et al. (1999). Reducing obesity via a school-based interdisciplinary intervention among youth: Planet Health. *Archives of Pediatrics and Adolescent Medicine, 153*, 409–418.

Hanevold, C., Waller, J., Daniels, S., Portman, R., & Sorof, J. (2005). The effects of obesity, gender, and ethnic group on left ventricular hypertrophy and geometry in hypertensive children: A collaborative study of the International Pediatric Hypertension Association. *Pediatrics, 113*, 328–333.

Harrell, J. S., McMurray, R. G., Bangdiwala, S. I., Frauman, A. C., Gansky, S. A., & Bradley, C. B. (1996). Effects of a school-based intervention to reduce cardiovascular risk factors in elementary-school children: The cardiovascular health in children (CHIC) study. *The Journal of Pediatrics, 128*, 797–805.

Jahns, L., Siega-Riz, A. M., & Popkin, B. M. (2001). The increasing prevalence of snacking among US children from 1977 to 1996. *Journal of Pediatrics,138*, 493–498.

Jelalian, E., Wember, Y. M., Bungeroth, H., & Birmaher, V. (2007). Practitioner review: Bridging the gap between research and clinical practice in pediatric obesity. *Journal of Child Psychology and Psychiatry, 48*, 115–127.

Kimm, S., Glynn, N. W., Kriska, A. M., Fitzgerald, S. L., Aaron, D. J., Similo, S. L., et al. (2000). Longitudinal changes in physical activity in a biracial cohort during adolescence. *Medicine & Science in Sports & Exercise, 32*, 1445–1454.

LeMura, L. M., & Maziekas, M. T. (2002). Factors that alter body fat, body mass, and fat-free mass in pediatric obesity. *Medicine & Science in Sports & Exercise, 34*, 487–496.

Luepker, R. V., Perry, C. L., McKinlay, S. M., Nader, P. R., Parcel, G. S., Stone, E. J., et al. (1996). Outcomes of a field trial to improve children's dietary patterns and physical activity: The Child and Adolescent Trial for Cardiovascular Health (CATCH). *JAMA, 275*, 768–776.

Manios, Y., Moschandreas, J., Hatzis, C., & Kafatos, A. (2002). Health and nutrition education in primary schools of Crete: Changes in chronic disease risk factors following a 6-year intervention programme. *British Journal of Nutrition, 88*, 315–324.

Manson, J. E., Nathan, D. M., Krolewski, A. S., Stampfer, M. J., Willett, W. C., & Hennekens, C. H. (1992). A prospective study of exercise and incidence of diabetes among US male physicians. *Journal of the American Medical Association, 268*, 63–67.

Manson, J. E., Rimm, E. B., Stampfer, M. J., Colditz, G. A., Willett, W. C., Krolewski, A. S., et al. (1991). Physical activity and incidence of non-insulin dependent mellitus in women. *Lancet, 338*, 774–778.

Must, A., & Strauss, R. S. (1999). Risks and consequences of childhood and adolescent obesity. *International Journal of Obesity Related Metabolic Disorders, 23*, S2–S11.

Nemet, D., Barkan, S., Epstein, Y., Friedland, O., Kowen, G., & Eliakim, A. (2005). Short- and long-term beneficial effects of a combined dietary-behavioral-physical activity intervention for the treatment of childhood obesity. *Pediatrics, 115*, 443–449.

Nicklas, T. A., Demory-Luce, D., Yang, S. J., Baranowski, T., Zakeri, I., & Berenson, G. (2004a). 1973–1994: The Bogalusa Heart Study. *Journal of American Dietetic Association, 104*, 1127–1140.

Nicklas, T. A., Elkasabany, A., Srinivasan, S. R., & Berenson, G. S. (2001). Trends in nutrient intake of 10-year-old children over two decades (1973–1994): The Bogalusa Heart Study. *American Journal of Epidemiology, 153*, 969–977.

Nicklas, T. A., Morales, M., Linares, A., Yang, S. J., Baranowski, T., De Moor, C., et al. (2004b). Children's meal patterns have changed over a 21-year period: The Bogalusa Heart Study. *Journal of American Dietetic Association, 104*, 753–761.

Ogden, C. L., Carroll, M. D., Curtin, L. R., McDowell, M. A., Tabak, C. J., & Flegal, K. M. (2006). Prevalence of overweight and obesity in the United States, 1999–2004. *Journal of American Medical Association, 295*, 1549–1555.

Pate, R. R., Pratt, M., Blair, S. N., Haskell, W. L., Macera, C. A., & Bouchard, C. (1995). Physical activity and public health. A recommendation from the Centers for Disease Control and Prevention and the American College of Sports Medicine. *Journal of American Medical Association, 273*, 402–407.

Pate, R. R., Ward, D. S., Saunders, R. P., Felton, G., Dishman, R. K., & Dowda, M. (2005). Promotion of physical activity in high school girls: A randomized controlled trial. *American Journal of Public Health, 95*, 1582–1587.

Prochaska, J. J., & Sallis, J. F. (2004). A randomized controlled trial of single versus multiple health behavior change: Promoting physical activity and nutrition among adolescents. *Health Psychology, 23*, 314–318.

Sääkslahti, A., Numminen, P., Salo, P., Tuominen, J., Helenius, H., & Välimäki, I. (2004). Effects of a three-year intervention on children's physical activity from age 4 to 7. *Pediatric Exercise Science, 16*, 167–80.

Saelens, B. F., Sallis, J. F., Wilfey, D. E., Patrick, K., Cella, J. A., & Buchta, R. (2002). Behavioral weight control for overweight adolescents initiated in primary care. *Obesity Research, 10*, 22–32.

Sallis, J. F., McKenzie, T. L., Conway, T. L., Elder, J. P., Prochaska, J. J., Brown, M., et al. (2003). Environmental interventions for eating and physical activity: A randomized controlled trial in middle schools. *American Journal of Preventive Medicine, 24*, 209–217.

Salmon, J., Booth, M. L., Phongsavan, P., Murphy, N., & Timperio, A. (2007). Promoting physical activity among children and adolescents. *Epidemiological Reviews, 29*, 144–159.

Savoye, M., Shaw, M., Dziura, J., Tamborlane, W. V., Rose, P., Guandalini, C., et al. (2007). Effects of a weight management program on body composition and metabolic parameters in overweight children: A randomized controlled trial. *JAMA, 297*, 2967–2704.

Snethen, J. A., Broome, M. E., & Cashin, S. E. (2006). Effective weight loss for overweight children: A meta-analysis of intervention studies. *Journal of Pediatric Nursing, 21*, 45–56.

Stice, E., Shaw, H., & Marti, C. N. (2006). A meta-analytic review of obesity prevention programs for children and adolescents: The skinny on interventions that work. *Psychological Bulletin, 132*, 667–691.

Taylor, R. W., McAuley, K. A., Barbezat, W., Strong, A., Williams, S. M., & Mann, J. I. (2007). APPLE Project: 2-y findings of a community-based obesity prevention program in primary school-age children. *American Journal of Clinical Nutrition, 86*, 735–742.

Taylor, W. C., & Sallis, J. F. (1997). Determinants of physical activity in children. In A. P. Simopoulos & K. N. Pavlou, (Eds.), *Nutrition and fitness: Metabolic and behavioral aspects in health and disease* (pp. 159–167). Washington, DC: American Psychological Association.

Thomas, H. (2006). Obesity prevention programs for children and youth: Why are their results so modest? *Health Education Research, 21*, 783–795.

Tsiros, M. D., Sinn, N., Coates, A. M., Howe, P. R. C., & Buckley, J. D. (2008). Treatment of adolescent overweight and obesity. *European Journal of Pediatrics, 167*, 9–16.

US DHHS. (1999). *Child health USA.* Rockville, MD: Human Services.

US DHHS. (2000). *Healthy People 2010: Understanding and improving health*, (2nd ed.). Washington, DC: U.S. Government Printing Office.

van Sluijs, E. M. F., McMinn, A. M., & Griffin, S. J. (2008). Effectiveness of intervention to promote physical activity in children and adolescents: Systematic review of controlled trials. *British Medical Journal, 335*, 703–715.

Wabitsch, M. (2000). Overweight and obesity in European children: definition and diagnostic procedures, risk factors and consequences for later health outcome. *European Journal of Pediatrics, 159*, S8–S13.

Wadden, T. A., Stunkard, A. J., Rich, .L, Rubin, C. J., Sweidwl, G., & McKinney, S. (1990). Obesity in black adolescent girls: A controlled clinical trial of treatment by diet, behavior modification, and parental support. *Pediatrics, 85*, 345–352.

Part II
Treating Obesity in the Adult and Elderly Populations

Chapter 6
Why Do Some People Lose Weight and Keep It Off? Ten Common Steps for Successful Weight Loss Over the Lifespan

Larry C. James

The health and psychological consequences of weight problems and obesity have been well documented over the past 30 years. Pi-Sunyer (1991) and Van Itallie (1985) documented more than 15–20 years ago the adverse effects of obesity. Wadden and Stunkard (2002), Baum, Revenson, and Singer (2001), Manson et al. (1995), Foster, Wadden, Kendall, Stunkard, and Vogt (1996), and Fairburn and Brownell (2005) have all eloquently described the health consequences of obesity. These authors have provided data to document that as one's weight increases beyond a body mass index (BMI) of 27, morbidity increases as well as diabetes, cancer, essential hypertension, depression, orthopedic problems, negative self-image, and a sense of worthlessness and medical complications from cholesterol disorders.

Needless to say, the obesity research data shown above suggest that it is rather unlikely for an obese patient to lose weight and keep it off. Yet, some researchers have implemented interventions or described key components to successful weight loss (Epstein, Valoski, Wing, & McCurley 1994; Epstein, 1996; Perri, Nezu, & Viegener, 1992; Perri, Shapiro, Ludwig, Twentyman, & McAdoo, 1984; Wing, 2002). How do some patients lose weight and maintain the weight loss for life and others are usually unsuccessful? Are there common aspects to successful weight loss across the lifespan?

James and his colleagues in 1995 at Tripler Army Medical Center sought to develop a healthy lifestyle treatment program for patients diagnosed with obesity, type II diabetes, essential hypertension, and elevated cholesterol (≥ 200). James, Folen, Garland, and Davis (1997a) and James et al. (1997b) built their program on the years of successful obesity research programs pioneered by Wing (1997), Perri et al. (1984, 1992), Wadden and Stunkard (2002), and Brownell and Jeffrey (1987). James and Folen integrated these research findings into their healthy lifestyle program. James and Folen's healthy lifestyle program has been providing cutting-edge services to obese patients since 1995 and has provided services to over 1000 male and female patients. In 1997, James and Folen et al. published their findings that summarized the common variables for successful weight loss in both male and female adult patients. These researchers identified 10 variables for successful weight loss based on their data. James, Folen, and Earles (2001) and James, Folen, and Noce (1998) later expanded their program to include innovative telemedicine technology to deliver clinical services to a greater number of patients throughout the Pacific Rim (Earles, James, Folen, & Verschell, 2001; James, Folen, & Earles, 2001). Not only did

L.C. James (✉)
Department of Psychology, Tripler Army Medical Center, Tripler Army Medical Center, Tripler AMC, Honolulu 96859, HI, USA
e-mail: JamesBDaddy@Aol.Com

L.C. James, J.C. Linton (eds.), *Handbook of Obesity Intervention for the Lifespan*, DOI 10.1007/978-0-387-78305-5_7, © Springer Science+Business Media, LLC 2009

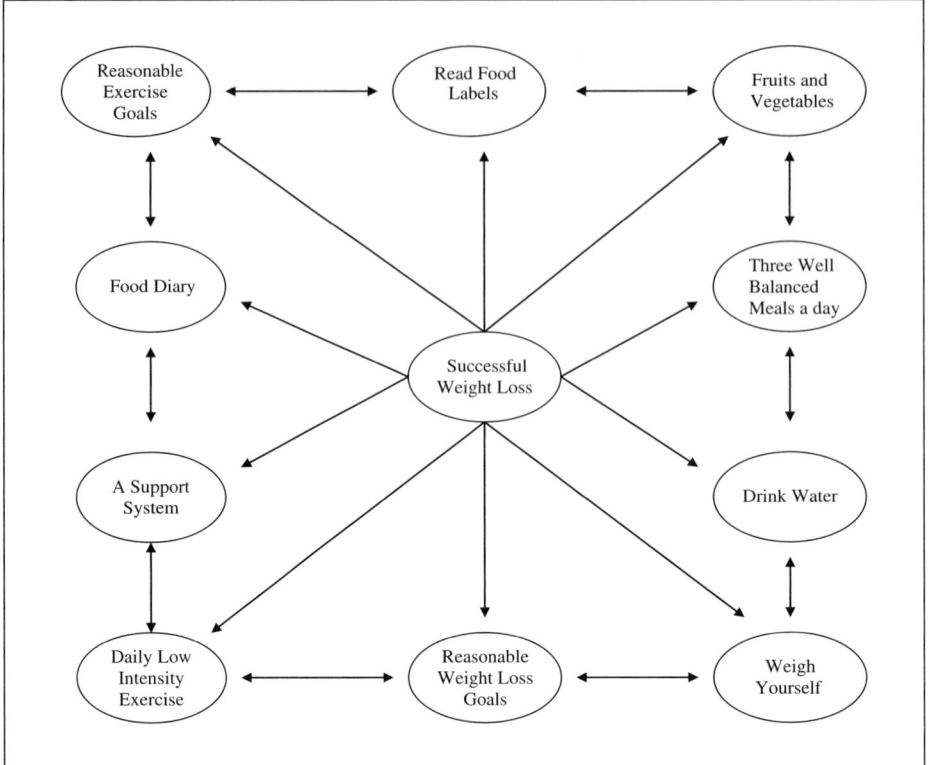

Fig. 6.1 Essential components of successful long term weight loss

these researchers use innovative technology to expand their services, but they also documented treatment efficacy in a male-minority population (1998).

In this chapter, the author will draw from the research of James et al. (1997a, 1997b, 1999, 2001) as well as the findings of the many researchers discussed above to provide the reader with an understanding of the essential components to successful, long-term weight loss.

Figure 6.1 illustrates the 10 essential components to successful weight loss. In Fig. 6.1, the author exhibits the circular manner in which these 10 variables are inter-connected and related, each variable driving the other. None of these variables can maintain weight loss completely on its own. Figure 6.1 yields the complex behavioral components that require lifelong support and commitment to the weight-loss journey.

Daily, Low-Intensity Exercise

Our patients arrive at treatment programs around the country with great enthusiasm, excitement and energy, determined *THIS TIME* to lose around 50 lb in 2 weeks and keep the weight off. Unfortunately, the vast majority of our patients will not only regain the 50 lb, but most likely additional weight also. Why? We have found that the major hurdle for patients is the "burden of exercise" as a patient once phrased it. Why the "burden"? Exercise is usually seen as a burden because in the United States the majority of Americans do not understand important aspects about the physiology of weight loss. For example, most of our patients have no real understanding of their target heart rate and, perhaps more importantly, most of our patients were taught the myth of "no pain no gain" when it comes to weight-loss exercise.

Jakicic, Wing, Butler, and Robertson (1995) pioneered what is now referred to as "short bouts of exercise." In their 1995 paper entitled *Prescribing Exercise in Multiple "Short Bouts Versus One Continuous Bout,"* they found that women participating in the short bout of exercise did statistically better than women enrolled in the long bout of exercise to lose weight. In other words, these researchers demonstrated that two 20-min periods of exercise was far better than one continuous 40-min long bout of exercise.

We found that in our program at Tripler Army Medical Center, the more a patient's weight exceeded 200 lb, the higher the likelihood that short bouts of exercise would work. Why? There were three very practical reasons. First, the patients did not get injured. Obese patients could tolerate walking for 20 min twice a day without experiencing an injury. Second, obese patients have paired exercise with pain over the years, and we found that the word exercise, although spelled differently, meant pain to our patients. Thus, they would try to lose weight without exercise. The psychological aspect of pain was a major deterrent for our patients. Once patients learned that he/she could exercise for two 20-min periods and the weight-loss benefits would be equal to, if not better than, the continuous 40-min bout of exercise, they become motivated to exercise. Even better, 20-min exercise periods would not hurt their bodies. The third factor was the variable *time*. Particularly for female patients, it was reported that they could easily find the time to exercise for two 20-min periods each day and still manage their house. A patient once said that a 40-min exercise period really equaled 2 h. She explained that it would take 30 min to get to the gym, 40 min to exercise, and at east 30 min to arrive back at home and shower – she did not have an extra 2 h in her day.

We have emphasized not only a short bout of exercise for patients but also doing it *daily* as well. We have found that in order for obese patients to be successful at weight, it must be done daily. Most obese patients arrived at their current weight because they were unsuccessful at the well-disciplined routine of trying to exercise every Monday, Wednesday, and Friday at 5:30 p.m. for 1 h; it just won't work. Therefore, to be successful, we have found that exercise has to be incorporated into the patient's daily lifestyle routine.

Weigh Yourself

Because of how the body's fat cells work, it is very difficult to lose weight and maintain the weight loss without being weighed at least twice a week. Our patients simply do not understand the physiology of fat cells and all too often try to avoid being weighed. We know that our patients avoid being weighed because of the depressive cycle of seeing the scale move upward rather than downward. Clearly, our long-term data suggest that weighing oneself at least twice a week is common among patients who successfully manage their weight.

Reasonable Weight-Loss Goals

The example of a patient gaining 50 lb rather than losing 50 lb was given earlier. Frequently, our patients set goals that are unrealistic such as losing 50 lb in a 2-week program, and of course, gaining more weight than he/she lost is the normal process.

Setting reasonable weight-loss goals that are obtainable each week has shown to be very successful over the past 10 years in our program. The goal standard of a 10% weight lost is seen as ideal, but perhaps an overall long-term, goal. In our program, we have learned that the thought of a 10% weight loss, and maintaining the weight loss, can be intimidating. Thus, we ask patients to lose 1 lb/week, a goal easily obtainable. Why this strategy? Our obese patients have been unsuccessful for many years, and once they experience the steady success of a 1-lb/week weight loss, it motivates these patients rather than trigger the depression associated with unsuccessful weight loss. Usually, patients would say, "doctor, 1 lb a week is nothing, I want to lose 10 lb a week." Eventually the patients realize the 10-lb/week weight-loss strategy has not served them well in the past and they welcome this new strategy as well as its success. Moreover, 1 lb/week equals 4 lb/month. Patients who maintain this rate of weight loss find that at the 10-month mark, he/she has lost 20–40 lb.

Reasonable Exercise Goals

Common among those who wish to lose weight is the frequent unreasonable exercise goal. Many of the obese patients have lived sedentary lifestyles for at least the past decade and now set a goal of running 5 miles each day. Failure at this exercise goal is usually followed by disappointment, the shame of being unsuccessful once again, perhaps depression and then more weight gain. We have had success with our patients setting an exercise goal that is very easy to obtain and does not involve pain, only success. For example, we encourage the patient who hasn't exercised in years to walk to the end of the block as an exercise goal. Thereafter, we add an additional block each week. We ask our patients to select an exercise that is doable so that he/she can experience some success at exercise. The end result is that the patient will have the motivation to do more exercise.

Three Well-Balanced Meals Each Day

Diets and quick remedies are a part of a 4-billion-dollar weight-loss industry. Yet, the success and utility of the fad and quick weight-loss fixes lack the science to support its efficacy. Thus, we teach patients that eating three well-balanced meals each day is the ideal way for them to consume meals. We have found that most of our patients say to themselves, "I want to lose weight, so I should only eat once a day."

A nutritionist teaches the patients about fat cells and that their bodies assume that they're starving when consuming only one meal a day. As a result, their metabolism will slow down because it assumes the person is starving. We know that this slows down the weight-loss process. Most patients have a hard time comprehending that they actually have to eat well-balanced meals if they want to acquire long-term weight loss.

Drink Water

Most who struggle with their weight may unconsciously believe that sports drinks are a staple of a well-balanced diet. Or the sports drink that has 400 times the normal daily vitamin requirement for vitamin C is 400 times better for their weight loss – it's not. Most Americans do not realize that the humane body was not designed to consume anything but regular water. The closer a patient can consume just plain water, the higher the likelihood the weight-loss efforts will come easier.

Consume Fruits and Vegetables

A male patient was once asked what are the basic food groups? He replied "well Doctor, you have the pizzas, the beers, cold cuts your donut snack food group." Unknowingly, many of our patients are not cognizant of the fact that fruits and vegetables are a necessary part of nutritional intake. Moreover, many green vegetables have natural anti-oxidants that help fight disease. We have found that, like increased water consumption, as the patients increases their fruits and vegetables, the easier it will be to maintain weight loss over time.

The Weight-Loss Diary

Most patients who struggle with their weight eat and buy food impulsively. They tend to under-report their food and calorie consumption by 30–50%. We require our patients to write down in a food diary everything that they eat and/or drink each day. There are many benefits to this technique. First, it slows down the impulsive eating behavior for a minute to allow the patient to assess the nutritional value of the item. Second, it provides a more accurate account of what the patient actually consumes each day. We have asked patients over the years what they most like and dislike about our program.

Unanimously, patients report that they dislike the daily requirement to maintain a food diary. Nevertheless, they all report the value of a food diary in helping them manage their weight.

Read Food Labels

Reading food labels goes hand-in-hand with keeping a food diary – both are essential. Most adults misperceive the true nutritional value of their food choices without reading the food labels. Thus, we have a registered dietitian teach classes on reading food labels. Patients tend to rely on the pastel colors and phrases such as "lite, low cal or reduced fat." Our dietitian teaches patients the actual meaning of these terms and how to ascertain if product A is actually healthier than product B.

A Support System and Family Involvement

Field, Barnoya, and Colditz (2002), Brownell and Jeffrey (1987), Wing (2002), Foster et al. (1996), and Klem et al. (1997) discuss the complicated array of emotions commonly associated with the difficult weight-loss journey for patients. These authors as well as others (Perri, Nezu, & Viegener, 1992; James et al., 1999; Perri et al., 1984; Wadden & Stunkard, 2002; Wing & Polley, 2001; Earles, 2007) discuss not only the role of emotions in successful weigh loss but also the need for a support group.

Epstein et al. (1994) conducted a 10-year longitudinal study with children and examined what were the positive impacts upon successful weight loss and described variables that increased outcome. In a later study, Epstein (1996) suggested that family support and a support system were critical to weight-loss outcome. In a similar manner, we have found that after 10 years of research, having a support system is critical to successful weight loss and weight-loss maintenance.

The following is a case illustration of the treatment provided to an obese, minority male patient with a complicated history. The case provides how the essential aspects of a successful weight-loss research were applied in a clinical setting.

Case Example

Tommy was a 26-year-old male of mixed Hawaiian, Filipino, and Samoan ethnic background. Tommy was self-referred to the Tripler Medical Center Healthy Lifestyle program after consultation with his family physician. Tommy's lipid panel, blood pressure, and weight combined were seen as life threatening. Tommy was 5′10″ in height and weighed 268 lb. His 23″ neck was coupled with a bulging and large midsection as well as a blood pressure of 160/110, a total cholesterol of 464, and a fasting glucose of 146. Tommy had been unsuccessful at many weight-loss attempts, fad, and starvation diets.

Additionally, Tommy felt that exercise would not help in his weight-loss efforts because he had a "bad back" and his "knees were shot." Exercise for Tommy was always a painful experience because he believed that "no pain no gain" was the correct model for an affective weight-loss strategy. He enrolled in the intensive 3-week day treatment program that includes weekly follow-up for 12 months after the completion of the 3-week program. The program's hallmarks are teaching patients to consume three healthy, well-balanced meals each day rather than fad diets, healthy food choices, and daily low-intensity exercise. A significant improvement for the patient was the weekly support group his spouse and three children attended. As a result of the support group, Tommy and his family began to exercise daily together and plan all meals. Initially, Tommy had a great deal of difficulty with low-intensity exercise. Likewise he did not understand the physiological benefits of walking rather than running, in particular, for a person of his size who had his physical limitations. Tommy was taught to set as a goal achieving 65–70% of his maximum heart rate while exercising. In addition, he was taught cognitive behavioral techniques in selecting meals and problem-solving emotional issues. Tommy began to go to grocery shop with a well-thought list rather than doing impulsive buying. The program's dietitian taught Tommy, his spouse, and children how to read food label as part of a grocery store field trip. He actively participated in the 3-week day treatment program and the yearlong weekly follow-up program. At 12 months post the start of treatment, Tommy's weight had decreased to 245 lb. His blood pressure had stabilized at 148/86 and his total cholesterol was reduced from 464 to 240 with a fasting glucose of 100. Tommy was successful at engaging his family in his daily evening exercise routine. Thus, his spouse and children began to lose weight as well.

Conclusion

Losing weight and maintaining the weight loss over time is a difficult and complex process. In this chapter the author provided 10 essential components that are required for patients to maintain a successful weight-loss pattern. These 10 essential components were drawn from over 10 years of clinical research in the authors' obesity treatment program as well as data from other successful programs around the country. We have found that daily, low-intensity exercise is the hallmark and cornerstone for any patient to lose and maintain their weight. This critical feature when coupled with the other nine essential components greatly increases the likelihood that patients will obtain long-term successful weight-loss management.

References

Baum, A., Revenson, T. A., & Singer, J. A. (2001). *Handbook of health psychology*. Mahwah, NJ: Lawrence Erlbaum Associates.

Brownell, K. D., & Jeffrey, R. W. (1987). Improving long-term weight loss: Pushing the limits of treatment. *Behavior Therapy, 18*, 353–374.

Earles, J., James, L. C., Folen, R. A., & Verschell, M. (2001). Incorporating behavioral telehealth in the treatment of obesity. *A poster presented at The American Psychological Convention*, August, San Francisco.

Earles, J. E., Kerr, B., James, L. C., & Folen, R.A. (2007). Clinical effectiveness of the LEAN Program: A military healthy lifestyle program. *Journal of Clinical Psychology In Medical Settings, 14*(1), 51–57.

Epstein, L. H. (1996). Family-based interventions for obese children. *International Journal of Obesity, 20*(Supp. 1), S14–S21.

Epstein, L. H., Valoski, A., Wing, R. R., & McCurley, J. (1994). Ten-year outcomes of behavioral family based treatment for childhood. *Health Psychology, 13*, 373–383.

Fairburn, C. G., & Brownell, K. D. (2005). *Eating disorders and obesity* (2nd ed.). New York: Guildford Press.

Field, A. E., Barnoya, J., & Colditz, G. A. (2002). Behavioral weight control. In T. A. Wadden & A. J. Stunkard (Eds.), *Handbook of obesity treatment* (pp. 3–18). New York: Guilford.

Foster, G. D., Wadden, T. A., Kendall, P. C., Stunkard, A. J., & Vogt, R. A. (1996). Psychological effects of weight-loss and regain: A prospective evaluation. *Journal of Consulting and Clinical Psychology, 64*(4), 752–757.

Jakicic, J. M., Wing, R. R., Butler, B. A., & Robertson, R. J. (1995). Prescribing exercise in multiple short bouts versus one continuous bout: Effects on adherence, cardio-respiratory fitness, and weight loss in overweight women. *International Journal of Obesity, 19*, 893–901.

James, L., Folen, R., Garland, F., & Davis, M. (1997a). New frontiers for clinical health psychology: Our leadership role in inpatient weight management programs. *Professional Psychology: Research & Practice, 28*(2), 146–152.

James, L., Folen, R. Garland, F., Noce, M., Edwards, C., Gohdes, D., et al. (1997b). The Tripler LEAN program: A healthy lifestyle model for the treatment of obesity. *Military Medicine, 162*, 328–332.

James, L. C., Folen, R. A., & Earles, J. (2001). Behavioral telehealth applications in the treatment of obese soldiers. *Journal of Military Psychology, 13*(3), 177–186.

James, L. C., Folen, R.A., & Noce, M. A. (1998). A healthy lifestyle program for the treatment of obesity in minority men. *Journal of Clinical Psychology in Medical Settings, 5*(3), 259–273.

James, L. C., Folen, R. A., Page, H., Noce, M., & Britton, C. (1999). The Tripler LEAN program: A two-year follow-up report. *Military Medicine, 164*(6), 389–395.

Klem, M. L., Wing, R. R., McGuire, M. T., Seagle, H. M., & Hill, J. O. (1997). A descriptive study of individuals successful at long-term maintenance of substantial weight-loss. *American Journal of Clinical Nutrition, 66*, 239–246.

Manson, J. E. Willett, W. C., Stampfer, M. J. Colditz, G. A., Hunter, D. J., Hankinson, S. E., et al. (1995). Body weight and mortality among women. *New England Journal of Medicine, 333*(11), 677–685.

Perri, M. G., Nezu, A. M., & Viegener, B. J. (1992). *Improving the long-term management of obesity*. New York: Wiley.

Perri, M. G., Shapiro, R. M., Ludwig, W. W., Twentyman, C. T., & McAdoo, W. G. (1984). Maintenance strategies for the treatment of obesity: An evaluation of relapse prevention training and post treatment contact by mail and telephone. *Journal of Consulting and Clinical Psychology, 52*, 404–413.

Pi-Sunyer, F. X. (1991). Health implications of obesity. *American Journal of Clinical Nutrition, 53*, 1595S–1603S.

Van Itallie, T. B. (1985). Health implications of overweight and obesity in the United States. *Annals of Internal Medicine, 103*, 983–988.

Wadden, T. A., & Stunkard, A. J. (2002). *Handbook of obesity treatment*. New York: Guilford.

Wing, R. R. (1997). Behavioral approaches to the treatment of obesity. In G. Bray, C. Bouchard, & P. T. James (Eds.), *Handbook of obesity* (pp. 855–873). New York: Marcel Dekker.

Wing, R. R. (2002). Behavioral weight control. In T. A. Wadden & J. Stunkard (Eds.), *Handbook of obesity treatment* (pp. 301–316). New York: Guilford.

Wing, R. R., & Polley, B. A. (2001). Obesity. In A. Baum, T. A. Revenson & J. E. Singer (Eds.), *Handbook of health psychology* (pp. 263–279). Mahwah, NJ: Lawrence Erlbaum Associates.

Chapter 7
Obesity and Older Adults: To Lose or Not to Lose???

Kristen H. Sorocco, Reginald Labossiere, and Karen M. Ross

Abstract The prevalence of obesity is increasing across all age cohorts including individuals aged 65 years and older. The purposes of this chapter are to provide an overview of the prevalence of obesity in older individuals, to review the adverse and beneficial health impacts of obesity as we age, and to provide treatment recommendations for obesity among older adults. Three cases using different treatment strategies will be discussed and patient resources will be provided.

Introduction

Until recently, it has been unclear whether or not it is in the patient's best interest to recommend weight loss to an older adult who meets criteria for being overweight or obese. The controversy stems from the natural changes in body weight and composition that occur with aging, beneficial effects of obesity among older adults, and limited research data. Villareal, Apovian, Kushner, and Klein (2005) provide a nice review of changes in body weight and composition across the lifespan. In general, aging is associated with a decrease in fat-free mass and an increase in fat mass until the age of 70, at which point in time both decline. This change in body composition is most likely a consequence of diminished physical activity rather than the aging process itself. There also is a redistribution of fat-free mass and fat mass as we age, with greater accumulation in the abdomen. Health benefits associated with obesity include an increased bone mineral density, and decreased osteoporosis, and hip fractures in older adults (For review see Villareal et al., 2005).

Further complicating the question of the benefits of weight-loss therapy to older adults is the paucity of research on obesity among older adults and the limitation of existing research by research design, often resulting in conflicting conclusions among studies. For example, cross-sectional population-based studies suggest that mean body weight and body mass index (BMI) gradually increase until about the age of 60 and then decline. However, longitudinal cohort studies suggest weight and BMI are relatively consistent or decrease only slightly with advanced age. In addition, there is very limited research data on the effectiveness of weight-loss programs for older adults.

Despite the limited research data, as the population of older adults continues to increase along with the prevalence of obesity, clinicians will need to appreciate the impact of obesity

K.H. Sorocco (✉)
Donald W. Reynolds Department of Geriatric Medicine, University of Oklahoma Health Sciences Center and VA Medical Center, Oklahoma City, OK 73104, USA
e-mail: Kristen-sorocco@ouhsc.edu

L.C. James, J.C. Linton (eds.), *Handbook of Obesity Intervention for the Lifespan*,
DOI 10.1007/978-0-387-78305-5_8, © Springer Science+Business Media, LLC 2009

on the health of older adults and how to best treat obesity among this age group. The purposes of this chapter are to provide an overview of the prevalence of obesity in older individuals, to review the adverse and beneficial health impacts of obesity as we age, and to provide treatment recommendations for obesity among older adults. Three cases using different treatment strategies will be discussed, and patient resources will be provided.

Definition of Obesity

Obesity simply defined is an excess of body fat (Villareal et al., 2005). There is not a quantitative definition of normal body fat. The association of body fat with disease depends on multiple factors like sex, gender, age, and fat distribution. The World Health Organization classifies body fat by using BMI: Normal weight is a BMI of 17–24, over-weight a BMI of 25–29, and obese a BMI of over 30. BMI is calculated by dividing the square of body weight in kilograms by the height in inches. This classification, even though based on large epidemiologic studies, gives a good estimate of the relation between body mass and disease. For example, one of the diagnostic criteria for metabolic syndrome includes body weight.

Prevalence of Obesity Among Older Adults

The prevalence of obesity is increasing across all age cohorts including individuals aged 65 years and older. In the later years of life, the prevalence of obesity rises and falls with age (Sezginsoy, Ross, Wright, & Bernard, 2004). Cross-sectional data reveals that obesity peaks in older individuals between 50 and 60 years of age and then declines between 60 and 80 years of age (Kennedy, Chokkalingham, & Srinivasan, 2004). Beyond the age of 80, there is a lower prevalence of obesity possibly due to earlier mortality from obesity-related illnesses, physiological anorexia of aging, and disease (Kotz, Billington, & Levine, 1999). However, even with the rise and fall of obesity across the lifespan, the National Center for Health Statistics (2004) found that between the ages of 65 and 74 years, 33% men and 39% women met criteria for obesity. With the increase in older citizens from the "Baby Boom" genera-tion, obesity will be a problem that will put a burden on an already saturated health-care system.

Adverse and Beneficial Effects of Obesity on Health of Older Adults

Obesity is associated with numerous chronic medical conditions and mortality (Refer to Table 7.1). Obesity-linked medical conditions include cardiovascular-related disorders, type 2 diabetes, arthritis, multiple cancers, gallbladder disease, osteoarthritis, asthma, sleep apnea, and depression (Sezginsoy, Ross, Wright, & Bernard, 2004). Obesity among older adults exacerbates normal age-related decline, decreasing physical functioning, and negatively influencing quality of life. Given the direct relationship between obesity and certain chronic medical conditions, obesity is associated with greater health service use and cost. However, there are limited data on the specific relationship between obesity and health service utilization among older adults.

The health benefits associated with obesity in older adults including improved bone health have been linked to an increase in hormonal secretion like estrogen, insulin, and leptin (Schindler, Ebert, & Friedrich, 1972; Reid, Evans, Cooper, Ames, & Stapleton, 1993; Thomas & Burguera, 2002). A key reason why these benefits are particularly significant is the high correlation between hip fractures and mortality. However, the benefits do not always outweigh the risks associated with obesity. In a recent position statement by the American Society for Nutrition and The Obesity Society, *weight-loss therapy that minimizes muscle and bone losses is recommended for older persons who are obese and who have functional impairments or medical complications that can benefit from weight loss* (Villareal et al., 2005).

Diagnosis of Obesity Among Older Adults

Aging is associated with a decrease in total energy expenditure while energy intake remains the same. This imbalance leads to accumulation of unhealthy fat. In older adults, age-related changes in body composition and loss of height, caused by compression fracture of vertebral bodies and kyphosis, alter the relation between BMI and percentage of body fat. So it is difficult to accurately measure body fat mass, because change in body composition in aging may underestimate the amount of fat, and also the change of height may over-estimate the percentage of fat.

Even though BMI is widely used, other methods to assess obesity include waist measurements, weight tables, subcutaneous fat measurement, and underwater weighing. Each of these methods has advantages and disadvantages (Sezginsoy, Ross, Wright, & Bernard, 2004). For example, waist measurements and weight tables do not require calculations but require either careful measurements or credible standards for older individuals (which are not available for those 75 years and older). A recent review of the literature determined that obesity among older adults can be diagnosed using standard clinical measures; however, BMI might have the most clinical utility (McTigue, Hess, & Ziouras, 2006).

Treatment of Obesity Among Older Adults

The treatment of obesity is a challenge, and the effectiveness of current treatment modalities among older adults is unclear. Weight loss in any age cohort improves obesity-related medical complications, physical functions, and quality of life. In young and middle-age adults, the goal of weight loss is more aimed at preventing medical complication, whereas in the elderly it is more to improve physical function and quality of life. Obesity can be managed by diet, exercise, drug treatment, surgery, behavioral modification, or any combination of these modalities. A recent review of the literature found that intensive counseling was successful in promoting modest sustained weight loss, but the jury is still out regarding the effectiveness of surgery or pharmacotherapy (McTigue, Hess, & Ziouras, 2006).

Diet

A realistic goal in the dietary management of obesity is to have the patient lose 5–10% of body weight and maintain this reduced weight. In prescribing a diet, it is important to choose one that the patient will comply with long enough to lose the necessary amount of weight, since most diets are not appetizing. Patients should reduce their diet by 500 calories a day to achieve 1–2 lb weight loss in 1 week. Weight loss naturally produces a decrease in energy expenditure because the body naturally adjusts for the decrease in intake. This creates a new balance between energy intake and utilization, often resulting in a plateau in weight loss. Increasing energy expenditure through exercise and strength training breaks the plateau by increasing metabolic rate. A balanced diet of over 1200 kcal usually provides enough vitamins and minerals, but adequate intake of vitamin D and calcium should be taken into consideration.

Exercise

Regular exercise is not essential for achieving initial weight loss, but it helps maintains weight loss. Data from the diabetes prevention program showed that at the end of 24 weeks, 60% of subjects who were 65 years and older met the 7% weight-loss goal compared with 43% of those who were less than 45 years old (Wing et al., 2004). These data suggest that for older adults, lifestyle therapy, including exercise, should be a primary treatment recommendation. Studies have shown that an increase in physical activity helps maintain weight loss. Exercise should promote expenditure of between 300 and 500 kcal/session, 3–4 times a week. Older patients should consult their physicians before starting an exercise program.

Medical

The data on utilization of medication in the older population is lacking because older individuals are often excluded in randomized trials. Given the multiple medications older adults are often prescribed, adding more for weight loss increases the risk of polypharmacy and chances for adverse side effects. There is also a financial consideration since most weight-loss drugs are not covered by Medicare or other insurance. Taking these factors into consideration, a BMI above 30 with an obesity-related medical complication or BMI more than 35 are indication for drug therapy by the FDA for all age groups.

Weight-Loss Drugs Work by Different Mechanisms

(1) Decreasing intake or increasing satiety. Sibutramine is the only drug in this category that was studied extensively. This drug causes weight loss by increasing satiation and decreasing food intake. Side effects are insomnia, constipation, and increased blood pressure and heart rate. Other drugs less used from that group are phentermine and mazindol. Ephedrine and caffeine are used in over-the-counter medication, but are not approved by the FDA. They work by increasing energy consumption and decreasing food intake.

(2) Blocking nutrient absorption. Orlistat is a pancreatic lipase inhibitor that decreases the absorption of fat and should be used with a low-fat diet to diminish flatulence and diarrhea. Patient taking this drug should be monitored for a liposoluble vitamin deficiency, and a vitamin supplement is recommended.

(3) By modulation of the central nervous system control of body weight. Leptin is an adipose-derived hormone, produced after eating. It is anti-obesity hormone in clinical trial.

Surgery

Surgery should be considered only in patients with morbid obesity, defined as a BMI between 35 and 39, with at least one severe obesity-related medical complications or a BMI greater than 40. Bariatric surgery is the most effective weight-loss therapy. The most common surgical procedures performed in the United States are the Roux-en-Y gastric bypass and the laparoscopic adjustable gastric band procedure. Studies in patients older than 60 have shown greater perioperative morbidity and mortality and modest weight loss or improvement of obesity-related medical complication compared with their younger counterparts (Sosa, Pombo, Pallavicini, & Ruiz-Rodriguez, 2004; Sugerman et al., 2004; St. Peter, Craft, Tiede, & Swain, 2005). Liposuction has been used to remove subcutaneous fat by aspiration under local anesthesia. This procedure can only remove a small amount of fat, making its use limited to cosmetic surgery. Older patients, in particular, need to have lifelong nutritional supplementation and medical follow-up, given the increased risks for nutritional deficiencies and complications associated with surgical procedures.

Psychological Interventions

There are a number of psychological interventions that can enhance the probability of treatment success for obesity among older adults. In particular, a number of cognitive behavioral therapeutic approaches (self-monitoring, goal setting, contingency management, stimulus control, and social support) can be used to facilitate a weight management program (Villareal, Apovian, Kushner, & Klein, 2005). Self-monitoring includes self-observation and self-recording of situational factors, thoughts, feelings, and behaviors associated with eating habits (Foreyt & Goodrick, 1993). For example, a food diary is a basic and useful tool to determine baseline eating patterns and intake as well as to track progress toward weight-loss goals. Patients are asked to keep a food diary for a week consisting of the times they eat, what they eat, how much they eat, and any other relevant environmental observations. The patterns from the food diary will identify possible treatment interventions such as the need for nutritional education, a dietician to alter the types of food a patient is eating, meals-on-wheels program, or social support and therapeutic recreation.

The data collected from self-monitoring also can assist in goal setting. As outlined by the Center for Disease Control and Prevention, goals need to be *s*pecific, *m*easureable, *a*ttainable, *r*elevant, and *t*ime based (SMART). Goals that focus on lifestyle changes rather than losing a specific amount of weight in a certain period of time are often more successful. Contingency management is a behavior modification technique that complements goal setting. Individuals are rewarded for reaching outlined goals. Contingency management is especially useful early on in weight management programs and to increase motivation to enhance readiness to change.

Stimulus control reduces environmental cues associated with maladaptive eating behaviors and increases the occurrence of behaviors that promote weight loss (Foreyt &

Goodrick, 1993). Examples include creating structured eating habits, such as planning out meals for the day, avoiding certain high-caloric foods such as soda, and scheduling times and locations of exercise. Similarly, activity scheduling could also be implemented during times when a patient is at the highest risk of overeating, such as late afternoon before dinner.

A key to any successful behavioral change is social support. This is especially true for older adults who are already at risk for a limited social support network. Therefore, encouraging older adults to identify a support person to help them reach their goals, find a support group for weight loss (such as a local gym with senior exercise programs, diabetes education group, Weight Watchers, etc.), or increase the contact by the physicians/treatment team through more frequent appointments or phone contacts would be beneficial. Working with an interdisciplinary treatment team alone will automatically enhance the amount of social support the older adult will receive to help them reach their weight-loss goals. Key disciplines to involve in the treatment plan beyond the physician might include a psychologist, social worker, dietitian, occupational therapist, and exercise specialist.

General Recommendations

Although there is some debate in the literature about the benefits of weight loss for obesity among older adults, there seems to be substantial evidence to promote weight-loss therapies that minimize muscle and bone loss for obese older adults (McTigue, Hess, & Ziouras, 2006). The prescription of weight-loss therapies should be dependent on the individual patient and his/her personal risk for or diagnosis of certain chronic diseases. Villareal, Apovian, Kushner, & Klein (2005) recommend a through medical history, physical examination, appropriate laboratory tests, review of medications, and assessment of readiness to lose weight before any weight-loss therapy is prescribed.

An initial comprehensive examination will help to identify the older obese patients who will most benefit from a weight-loss therapy. Inelmen and colleages (2003) suggest that patients in whom BMI values fall in the overweight range should only be counseled to lose weight if they are under the age of 70. For older individuals free of chronic disease with limited health risks, doctors should consider counseling patients to simply maintain their current weight. Older individuals with high cardiovascular risk are most likely to benefit substantially from weight-loss therapies (McTigue, Hess, & Ziouras, 2006). Finally, psychological approaches supporting lifestyle changes appear to have the most evidence of treatment success among older adults and therefore should be combined with any other weight-loss treatment modality.

Case Studies

When an older adult with obesity comes into the office, an initial question for providers to ask is "What health conditions does this patient's obesity either place him/her at risk for or how does it affect existing conditions?" Table 7.1 lists the medical conditions that are significantly influenced by weight loss. Below are three cases in which the above question was asked and the outcomes based on weight-loss interventions.

Table 7.1 Medical conditions significantly influenced by weight loss

Medical condition	Benefit of weight loss
Diabetes mellitus type II	Weight loss has been found to be more effective than drug therapy and more effective in the older adult population in prevention of diabetes.
Hypertension	Weight loss leads to lower blood pressure.
Hyperlipidemia	Leads to lower cholesterol levels.
Metabolic syndrome	Obesity increases the risk for this syndrome.
Obstructive sleep apnea	Obesity increases the risk for obstructive sleep apnea, and weight loss is key in the management of sleep apnea.
Osteoarthritis	Obesity increases the risk for osteoarthritis.

Case #1

Husband and wife were both diagnosed as obese, were prescribed weight loss, and weight loss was achieved.

Wife: 66 years old with a problem list that included hyperlipidemia, HTN on pharmacotherapy, osteoarthritis for which she needed analgesics, and chronic low back pain. Weight was 196 (BMI = 32.6). At f/u visit, she was found to have elevated triglycerides of over 500 and weight was up to 207 (BMI = 34.4). (She was also having compliance issues with antihypertensive therapy.) She was counseled at this visit about metabolic syndrome and her *urgent* need to get her weight, cholesterol, and blood pressure better controlled. At a follow-up 6 months later, her weight was down by nearly 20–188 lb (BMI = 31). She described a significant reduction in knee and back pain and did not require analgesics routinely any longer. Her triglycerides were much improved but she still required pharmacotherapy to get them at goal. At follow-up 6 months later, her weight was down by an additional 15 lb (173 lb; BMI = 28.8). She was elated at her and her husband's weight-loss success and reported it was much easier to lose weight with someone else.

Husband: 77 years old with a weight of 263 (BMI = 40) and had co-morbid conditions of hypertension, hyperlipidemia for which he was on pharmacotherapy, chronic low back pain, and obstructive sleep apnea. At a subsequent visit, his weight was 259 but he complained of right-sided hip pain. A radiograph taken was consistent with arthritis with joint space narrowing. At f/u appointment in May 2005, his weight was down by 15 lb to 244 (BMI = 37), but 6 months later his weight was up to 258 and reported he was no longer walking as he had been doing before. Six months later his weight was up to 268 (BMI = 40.7), and he admitted that his portion size was too large and was still sedentary. He was counseled extensively about his risk factors for heart disease, stroke, and functional loss and was referred to nutritionist and short-term goals of weight loss of 2 lb/week, walking everyday on treadmill, healthier snacks and breakfast, and one-fourth plate rule at supper. Six months later his weight was 227 lb (BMI = 34.5), down by 41 lb, and he reported that overall he was feeling much better (energy level was improved, his breathing was easier), but persistent hip pain led to an orthopedic referral and subsequent total hip replacement. At a follow-up 6 months later, the patient had lost an additional 27 lb (weight = 200 lb, BMI = 30.4), he was pain free and walked regularly on his treadmill, and his blood pressure was running so much lower that he was able to get off a medication.

Take-home points

Keys for the weight-loss success in this couple included social support, physician counseling, motivated patients, and referral to a nutritionist.

Case #2

An older adult who was diagnosed as obese was recommended weight loss, lost weight, and then regained weight.

Mrs. M: At the initial visit her weight was 225 (BMI = 41). She was 76 years old and had diabetes, hyperlipidemia, and CAD s/p stent placed a year prior. She was sedentary and so functionally compromised that the goal for physical activity made at that visit was for her to walk to the mailbox twice daily. She had chronic severe knee pain and had tried scheduled Tylenol and NSAIDs with incomplete relief and so she was prescribed a low dose of narcotic. Over the next 2 years, her weight went up and down by 15–20 lb. At follow-up appointment, her weight was 212, down by 34 lb from her highest weight, and her pain complaints were much improved. She was not requiring analgesics and was using a stationary bicycle 15 min a day. One year later her weight was down to 182 (BMI = 33). Her energy level was much improved and functionally she was out doing more than she had done in years. At her last clinic visit, 6 months later, her weight was back up by 15 lb (BMI = 36) and was cautioned to not let her weight continue to increase.

Take-home points

Weight loss is a chronic disease and needs to be managed as a chronic medical condition. Weight gain after successful weight loss is an all-too-common scenario, which is why weight management needs to be a continuous and ongoing part of medical treatment.

Case #3

An older adult's obesity was treated using bariatric surgery.

Ms. A: At 73 years of age, in addition to obesity, her problem list included chronic low back pain and spinal stenosis, fatty liver, osteoarthritis s/p bilateral knee replacements, and hyperlipidemia. Her weight was 221 and BMI = 39. Over the next several years she battled depression, chronic pain, and fatigue and her weight increased to 248 (BMI = 44). She then decided to meet with a surgeon who specialized in weight-loss surgery to discuss a surgical approach for her obesity. After meeting with the surgeon, she began saving money to cover the costs her insurance would not for the surgery. Nearly a year later she underwent gastric bypass surgery and at the last clinic visit her weight was 219 lb, down by 35 lb from her maximum weight (BMI = 38.8). She stated her functional level was the best it had been in years. She had previously described being unable to fix her hair due to fatigue and weakness in her upper extremities and would have to do it in stages. Now she was able to complete this important personal care without difficulty. Her breathing was much improved and she was able to get up on a small foot stool and change a light bulb, something she said she could have never had managed before the surgery. She was looking forward to starting a water-based exercise program once her scars were healed. Her cholesterol was so low that her medication was stopped.

Take-home points

Some *select* patients may benefit from surgical intervention as a last resort. Certainly, it is too early to see what the long-term effects are going to be with this patient.

Patient Resources

National Institutes of Health Exercise for Seniors webpage: Provides an overview and links to NIH publications from the National Institutes of Aging and National Institutes of Diabetes and Digestive and Kidney Diseases on exercise tips for older adults.
Web address: health.nih.gov/result.asp/244

Young at Heart: Tips for Older Adults: Publication from the National Institutes of Diabetes and Digestive and Kidney Disease on healthy eating and physical activity across your lifespan.
Web address: win.niddk.nih.gov/publications/young_heart.htm

Exercise: A Guide from the National Institutes on Aging: A publication to encourage exercise among older adults, promoting safety and motivation.
Web address: www.nia.nih.gov/HealthInformation/Publications/ExerciseGuide/

Physical Activity for Everyone: Are There Special Recommendations for Older Adults: A comprehensive website by the Centers for Disease Control and Prevention on exercise recommendations for older adults, strength training programs for older adults, and motivational and goal-setting tools. www.cdc.gov/nccdphp/dnpa/physical/recommendations/older_adults.htm

NIH Senior Health: An interactive website by the National Institutes on Aging to assist older adults when beginning an exercise program.
Web address: nihseniorhealth.gov/exercise/toc.html

References

Foreyt, J.P., & Goodrick, G.K. (1993). Evidence for success of behavior modification and weight loss and control. *Annals of Internal Medicine, 119* (7 Part 2), 698–701.

Inelmen, E.M., Sergi, G., Coin, A., Miotto, F., Peruzza, S., & Enzi, G. (2003). Can obesity be a risk factor in elderly people? *Obesity Reviews, 4,* 147–155.

Kennedy, R., Chokkalingham, K., & Srinivasan, R. (2004). Obesity in the elderly: Who should we be treating, and why, and how? *Current Opinion in Clinical Nutrition and Metabolic Care, 7,* 3–9.

Kotz, C.M., Billington, C.J., & Levine, A.S. (1999). Obesity and aging. *Clinics in Geriatric Medicine, 15* (2), 391–412.

McTigue, K.M., Hess, R. & Ziouras, J. (2006). Obesity in older adults: A systematic review of the evidence for diagnosis and treatment. *Obesity, 14* (9), 1483–1497.

National Center for Health Statistics (2004). Health, United States, 2004, with Chartbook on Trends in the Health of Americans. Hyattsville, MD: U.S. Department of Health and Human Services, Centers for Disease Control and Prevention.

Reid, I.R., Evans, M.C., Cooper, G.J., Ames, R.W., & Stapleton, J. (1993). Circulating insulin levels are related to bone density in normal postmenopausal women. *American Journal of Physiology, 265* (4 Pt 1), E655–9.

Schindler, A.E., Ebert, A., & Friedrich, E. (1972). Conversion of androstenedione to estrone by human tissue. *Journal of Clinical Endocrinology Metabolism, 35* (4):627–30.

Sezginsoy, B., Ross, K., Wright, J.E., & Bernard, M.A. (2004). Obesity in the elderly: Survival of the fit or fat. *Journal of the Oklahoma State Medical Association, 97* (10), 437–442.

Sosa, J.L., Pombo, H., Pallavicini, H., & Ruiz-Rodriguez, M. (2004). Laparoscopic gastric bypass beyond age 60. *Obesity Surgery, 14* (10):1398–401.

St. Peter, S.D., Craft, R.O., Tiede, J.L., & Swain, J.M. (2005). Impact of advanced age on weight loss and health benefits after laparoscopic gastric bypass. *Archives of Surgery, 140* (2):165–8.

Sugerman, H.J., DeMaria, E.J., Kellum, J.M., Sugerman, E.L., Meador, J.G., & Wolfe, L.G. (2004). Effects of bariatric surgery in older patients. *Annals of Surgery, 240* (2):243–7.

Thomas, T., & Burguera, B. (2002). Is leptin the link between fat and bone mass? *Journal of Bone Mineral Research, 17* (9):1563–9.

Villareal, D.T., Apovian, C.M., Kushner, R.F., & Klein, S. (2005). Obesity in older adults: Technical review and position statement of the American Society for Nutrition and NAASO, The Obesity Society. *Obesity Research, 13* (11), 1849–1863.

Wing, R.R., Hamman, R.F., Bray, G.A., Delahanty, L., Edelstein, S.L., Hill, J.O., et al. (2004). Achieving weight and activity goals among diabetes prevention program lifestyle participants. *Obesity Research, 12* (9):1426–34.

Chapter 8
Low-Intensity Exercise as a Treatment Intervention in Obese Adults

Mark Verschell

This chapter presents a summary of low-intensity exercise as it pertains to the prescription of safe and effective treatment plans by obesity healthcare providers. At first thought, the prescription of *low*-intensity exercise might seem imprudent in comparison to commonly endorsed criteria of physical fitness, such as "the lifelong ability to perform moderate-to-vigorous levels of physical activity without experiencing excessive fatigue" (American College of Sports Medicine [ACSM], 1998). In fact, low-intensity exercise may, in some cases, prove insufficient for improving objective measures of cardiorespiratory fitness. For many patients, however, these are points of moot debate. Physical limitations and individual differences in exertion tolerance often preclude augmentation of exercise intensity as a productive target of treatment. Clinical obesity management therefore emphasizes the adoption of consistent and balanced health behaviors, including the progressive approximation of physical fitness goals, rather than the achievement of perfect nutrition or ultimate physical fitness, in order to help patients attain maximal benefit at the lowest risk. In this regard, low-intensity exercise serves as the "lowest common denominator" of clinically prescribed exercise plans. Fortunately, many health benefits can be achieved via lower intensity exercise if the frequency and duration of training are appropriately adjusted.

Vanguard Agencies for Physical Fitness and Health Policy

The exercise guidelines in this chapter are drawn primarily from public health policy statements and expert consensus recommendations drafted by the American College of Sports Medicine (ACSM), the Centers for Disease Control and Prevention (CDC), the American Heart Association (AHA), the International Association for the Study of Obesity (IASO), the United States Department of Health and Human Services (HHS), National Institutes of Health (NIH), Office of the Surgeon General (OSG), and the President's Council on Physical Fitness and Sports (PCPFS). Similar to other areas of behavioral science, exercise and health research produces some degree of divergent and conflicting results due to the difficulties of implementing rigorous experimental controls. However, the systematic evaluations performed by these agencies over the past 15 years have generated increasingly consistent physical activity recommendations with regard to

M. Verschell (✉)
Health Psychology Service, Department of Psychology, Tripler Army Medical Center, Honolulu, HI, USA
e-mail: mark.verschell@us.army.mil

L.C. James, J.C. Linton (eds.), *Handbook of Obesity Intervention for the Lifespan*,
DOI 10.1007/978-0-387-78305-5_9, © Springer Science+Business Media, LLC 2009

maintaining and improving health. Therefore, it seems reasonable to implement them as "best practice guidelines" for facilitating the clinical management of obesity and related lifestyle-influenced medical disorders. Due to be issued by the HHS Office of Disease Prevention and Health Promotion in late 2008 are the "Physical Activity Guidelines for Americans," touted as the first federal guidelines to focus on physical activity.

Health Outcomes

Despite the difficulties inherent to applying experimental design to study the health outcomes of human behavior, observational research evidence strongly supports the relationship between physical activity and the maintenance of bodily health. Exercise is associated with the development of strong muscles and bones and the prevention of cardiovascular disease, stroke, diabetes mellitus, osteoporosis, hypertension, dyslipidemia, and several types of cancer. Exercise is also beneficial for improving cognitive and emotional functioning, including recovery from stroke, dementia, depression, and anxiety. Current and future research efforts show strong promise for identifying the physiological mechanisms precipitating these health benefits, such as the facilitation of peripheral glucose transport and metabolism via the development of lean muscle mass.

Treatment Parameters

Certainly, behavioral modification is one of the primary goals of the obesity healthcare provider. For this reason, it will prove prudent to differentiate between the terms "physical activity" and "exercise." A physical activity is simply any voluntary bodily movement that precipitates skeletal muscle contraction and utilizes metabolic energy. Exercise refers to the performance of physical activities within the context of a defined *behavioral plan* for the purpose of achieving physical *fitness* and medical and mental *health*. Exercise prescription often uses these terms interchangeably with the understanding that the referenced physical activities are both planned and goal oriented.

"Physical fitness" is an evolving and multidimensional concept that is currently defined in terms of skill-related, health-related, and physiological components. Skill-related components include agility, balance, coordination, speed, power, and reaction time. Although these elements of fitness are typically of greater focus in fields stressing competitive motor-skills performance, balance and coordination are important treatment targets for patients who are older or who have significant physical limitations. In the field of clinical obesity management, the health-related components of physical fitness serve as the immediate targets of behavioral intervention, and the physiological components serve as the initial indicators of improvements in medical health. The health-related components of physical fitness are performance-based indicators that reflect the capacity to perform essential activities of daily living and to avoid diseases that are significantly influenced by sedentary lifestyles. These components include (1) cardiorespiratory fitness, (2) muscular strength and endurance, and (3) flexibility.[1] The physiological components of fitness represent the statuses of the biological systems that respond positively to consistent exercise behaviors and include indicators of (1) metabolic fitness (e.g., blood pressure, blood lipids, fasting blood glucose and glucose tolerance, blood indices of thrombosis and systemic inflammation, liver enzyme levels), (2) morphologic fitness (e.g., waist circumference, body fat percentage, regional body fat distribution), and (3) bone integrity (e.g., mineral density).

Health outcomes of exercise follow a dose–response relationship and accrue in relation to the volume-by-modality summation of physical fitness training, where modality refers to categories of exercise that correspond to the performance-based components of physical fitness. The four primary modalities are termed cardiorespiratory (aka endurance, aerobic) training, resistance (aka strength) training, flexibility training (aka stretching), and balance training. Volume and modality factors thus become the primary behavioral parameters of prescribed exercise plans, and collectively they are referred to as the "FITT Principle," which defines the frequency, intensity, time (i.e., duration), and type (i.e., modality) of exercise. One of the main objectives of exercise prescription is to help patients manipulate the FITT parameters to achieve "progressive overload," which describes the process whereby muscle tissue and other physiological systems increase in functional capacity and efficiency via repetitive and incremental exposure to physical stress. In terms of overall health benefits, there are clearly many successful permutations of the FITT parameters. In fact, since all bodily movements simultaneously work our muscles and cause an increase in the amount of oxygen, nutrients, and neural signals flowing to them, overlap does occur across the training modalities. Generally, however, improvements in physical fitness (i.e., the "training effect") are relatively *specific* to the type of physical activity performed and the muscle groups involved. Interestingly, genetic and health status factors may precipitate significantly different responses to the same type and intensity of physical activity across individuals. Balanced exercise prescription should therefore incorporate a sufficient volume of training across a variety of activities within each training modality in order to achieve a breadth of favorable health outcomes. Patients who are training for performance-based fitness tests should also devote a sufficient quantity of training to the specific activities that will be tested.

In clinical practice, the obesity healthcare provider will frequently encounter patients who, at least initially, will not exceed the lower thresholds of exercise intensity and volume. In these situations, a stepwise approach to prescribing the various modalities of exercise is obviously warranted. Flexibility training is typically prescribed as the initial exercise modality, as it is an essential prerequisite for preventing injury, and requires relatively little time and physical exertion. Balance training can also be performed effectively at lower levels of physical exertion, but is usually prescribed after patients achieve consistency in performing rudimentary levels of cardiorespiratory training, due to its lack of influence on body weight and body composition. The reverse prescription pattern is sometimes appropriate for patients who are elderly, frail, medically compromised, or exceedingly unfit. Cardiorespiratory training is clearly the mainstay of exercise prescription for the treatment of obesity, since it is the modality with the largest effect on energy balance. Obesity practitioners should be cautious, however, to not eschew the prescription of resistance training, which not only improves muscular strength and endurance, but also contributes to the reduction of body fat and the development and maintenance of muscle mass.

Warm-Up, Flexibility, and Balance Training

All exercise sessions should be preceded by a period of warm-up that involves 5–10 min of low- and progressing-intensity large muscle activity using the same muscles and bodily motions that will be employed during subsequent training activities. Warm-up thus prepares the body for higher intensity exercise by increasing blood flow, body temperature, oxygen availability, and cellular metabolic rate. Flexibility training typically follows warm-up and involves stretching and range of motion activities to lengthen muscle fibers and lower their resting tension levels and increase connective tissue extensibility and joint function. "Static" stretching is performed by slowly lengthening the targeted muscle group to the end of its range of motion and holding the position for 15–30 s. This procedure is repeated 2–4 times for each targeted muscle group. Range of motion activities are performed similarly on the targeted joints, including the knees, ankles, hips, shoulders, and fingers. Flexibility training is, by nature, of relatively low intensity,[2] and research has shown that holding the end position of stretches for greater than 30 s provides little, if any, additional benefit. Progression is achieved primarily as a result of training consistency, and since the benefits of these activities appear to be relatively transient, they should be performed on most days in order to facilitate injury resistance, particularly for older patients and those with limited flexibility. Print and web-based resources for teaching patients stretching and range of motion exercises are widely available. Particularly helpful are free videos demonstrating chair-based flexibility exercises for patients with lower fitness levels, available from the National Center on Physical Activity and Disability (NCPAD) website.

Balance training is another form of low-intensity exercise that is typically prescribed for older patients, but is also appropriate for obese patients who are at risk for falling or who have difficulty moving between prone, sitting, and standing positions. Several types of physical activity have been used to improve muscular strength, neuromuscular coordination, and sensory feedback related to postural stability. These exercises teach patients to maintain stable body posture and to perform controlled bodily movements under a variety of conditions that necessitate good balance, including sitting and rolling on exercise balls, and changing leg positions while standing on foam pads. Training progression can be achieved by using increasingly unstable conditions and performing these activities with eyes closed. Research continues to accumulate regarding the most effective volumes of training to prevent balance-related injuries, but a good recommendation from the NCPAD calls for 2–3 repetitions of 8–10 exercises, to cover the major muscle groups and to be performed 2–3 days each week.

Cardiorespiratory Training

Cardiorespiratory activities are those that utilize large muscle groups in a continuous fashion, either rhythmically or dynamically. Tables listing the various types of endurance activities in conjunction with their average rate of energy expenditure are useful clinical tools, but skill level, personal interest, pain tolerance, and injury potential are also important considerations when prescribing these activities for the obese patient. In general, activities that involve competition, dynamic motion, and advanced skills demonstrate greater interindividual variation in energy expenditure. For example, racquetball has the potential for facilitating cardiorespiratory conditioning and weight loss, but patients with less skill or coordination may lose interest quickly if they cannot achieve a reasonable consistency of play. Conversely, highly skilled racquetball players may develop economy of motion that conserves energy expenditure relative to players with less skill.

The AHA and the American College of Sports Medicine published updated exercise guidelines for healthy adults in August 2007. These guidelines recommend moderate-intensity aerobic physical activity for a minimum of 30 min on 5 days each week or vigorous-intensity activity for a minimum of 20 min on 3 days each week. These recommendations are based on accumulating empirical evidence, suggesting that improvements in *cardio-respiratory fitness* are contingent upon training at moderate levels of intensity. Fortunately, a fair body of research has also demonstrated that reductions in body fat and total body mass, as well as improvements in medical health, can be achieved with frequent and extended periods of low-intensity cardiorespiratory training. In clinical obesity practice, aerobic exercise prescription targets progressive increments in total energy expenditure via manipulation of any of the FITT factors. Patients who can be reinforced to progressively increase cardiorespiratory training *intensity* may achieve additional health benefits, including improvements in oxygen delivery and consumption ($VO_{2\ max}$) and lactate threshold (LT) and greater risk reduction for chronic disease.

Intensity of Cardiorespiratory Training

$VO_{2\ max}$ and LT reflect the capacities of the cardiovascular and skeletal muscle systems to deliver oxygen to the working muscles, to transform food energy into metabolic energy via aerobic respiration, and to effectively process and remove metabolic waste products. Together, these measures describe the *rates* of non-sustainable maximum, and highest sustainable submaximum, energy expenditure; that is, how intense a person can exercise for brief and extended periods. Percentage $VO_{2\ max}$ and LT are typically measured by performance athletes to evaluate exercise intensity and the upper limits of exercise tolerance. However, these measures are rarely utilized in clinical obesity practice because they require a combination of ventilation volume and O_2/CO_2-sensing equipment or repetitive blood sampling and testing.

Heart rate (HR) has a relatively linear relationship with VO_2 and is therefore a useful method of gauging exercise intensity for patients who find the science of exercise physiology or the novelties of measuring cardiorespiratory fitness reinforcing (e.g., a HR wristwatch or armband monitor). Historically, exercise intensity has been expressed as a straight percentage of $VO_{2\ max\ (ml/kg/min)}$ and estimated using a straight percentage of $HR_{max\ (beats/min)}$ (i.e., 50–70% $VO_{2\ max}$ is approximately equal to 70–85% HR_{max}). More recent methods express exercise intensity as a percentage of the range of energy expenditure between resting metabolism and maximum utilization (i.e., oxygen uptake reserve [VO_2R]), yielding a better correlation between HR and VO_2 across the lower range of exercise intensities. Target HR is calculated using the Karvonen HR reserve method as (HRR × targeted % exercise intensity) + HR_{rest}, where $HRR = HR_{max} - HR_{rest}$. The traditional method of using age to estimate maximum HR (HR_{max} is approximately equal to 220 – age) is still employed routinely in clinical practice, despite its significant error of estimate (~10–12 bpm). The ASCM endorses the following VO_2R | HRR aerobic intensity classification system based on a 60-min exercise session: "Very light": <20%; "Light": 20–39%; "Moderate": 40–59%; "Hard": 60–84%; "Maximal": 100%.

A less demanding method of estimating cardiorespiratory exercise intensity involves subjective ratings of perceived exertion (RPE) and is preferred by a substantial percentage of obesity patients. These ordinal-level scales utilize effort-based anchors of increasing intensity and are influenced by physiological status and sensations (e.g., heart and respiration rate, blood pH and glucose levels, muscle lactic acid production, joint and muscle pain), psychological factors (e.g., mood, motivation, expectation, fatigue), and external variables related to the exercise environment (e.g., temperature, humidity, audiences). The Borg 15-point scale is perhaps the most empirically tested and clinically applied RPE scale of this type. In addition to being easy to understand, reliable, and simple to use, research has shown this scale to have good correlation with other physiological measures of work. The scale's numerical anchors range from 6 to 20 and correlate roughly with HR (divided by 10). Semantic anchors may be customized to include exercise examples relevant to the specific assessment context. The semantic anchors from Borg's standardized administration narrative translate generally as: "6": "no exertion at all"; "9": "very light exercise like walking"; "13": "somewhat heavy exercise but sustainable"; "17": "very strenuous exercise requiring extra effort to sustain"; and "19": "extremely strenuous exercise equivalent to the hardest ever experienced." Although an exercise test is the most accurate method to determine an activity-specific exercise prescription, there is general agreement that training ranges of 50–85% $VO_{2\ max}$ correspond to ratings of 12–16 on the $Borg_{6-20}$ scale.

Interestingly, research has suggested that the psychological and external RPE factors are more influential than the physiological factors at lower exercise intensities. This creates a therapeutic window for helping obesity patients to exercise more consistently and to progressively increase their energy expenditures. For example, exercise plans for patients who gravitate toward lower levels of exercise intensity may be modified to incorporate music, social distractions, and competitive play or to begin when temperatures are more conducive or when fatigue is less likely to be experienced. Adjusting these systems of reinforcement may help patients to perceive their levels of exertion to be lower than their physiological responses.

All of the previous measures, $\%VO_{2\ max}$, $\%HR_{max}$, $\%VO_2R$, $\%HRR$, and RPE, are *relative* indices of cardiorespiratory exercise intensity that describe an individual's rate of energy expenditure in relation to his/her level of cardiorespiratory fitness and body mass. Hence, they are useful for monitoring the achievement and progression of targeted intensity parameters. Another relative measure of cardiorespiratory exercise intensity encountered in clinical practice is the metabolic equivalent (MET), which defines an individual's rate of energy expenditure in relation to resting metabolic rate and body mass, that is, 1 MET = 3.5 $O_{2\ ml/kg/min}$. The MET is often used to categorize the different types of endurance activities according to their average rates of energy expenditure and hence is useful for helping patients to identify appropriate types of physical activity during the initial stages of behavioral planning. The MET is also used by healthcare policy agencies for defining cardiorespiratory energy expenditure targets for weight loss and body composition change. According to the most recent ACSM/AHA (2007) guidelines, "light," "moderate," and "vigorous" intensity activities are those involving less than three, three –six, and greater than six METs, respectively.

Training Volume and Progression Algorithm for Cardiorespiratory Fitness

The ACSM recommendations for healthy adults beginning a *moderate*-intensity exercise program progress from 6 weeks of initial conditioning involving 3–4 training sessions of 15–30 min at a rate of 40–60% HRR, to a 4–8 month improvement phase involving more rapid escalations in training volume, with the ultimate goal of achieving a maintenance phase involving 3–5 weekly training sessions of 20–60 min at a rate of 70–85% HRR. Although no specific system of low-intensity progression is outlined for deconditioned individuals, these guidelines provide an objective frame of reference from which clinicians can extrapolate endurance targets, based upon patients' individual levels of fitness and exertion tolerance. Daily volumes of physical activity can be accumulated using multiple bouts of shorter duration exercise, but each bout should endure for a minimum of 10 min in order to increase the likelihood of improving cardiorespiratory fitness. Of importance, these exercise guidelines are *in addition* to patients' routine activities of daily living, which are generally performed with light intensity when they endure for at least 10 continuous minutes.

Clinicians in obesity practice will undoubtedly encounter patients who require highly curtailed initial exercise plans and whose behaviors demonstrate limited capacity for progression.[3] Monitoring of cardiorespiratory fitness levels may prove to be a particularly reinforcing stimulus for these patients, as initial improvements tend to favor individuals with lower fitness levels and those who are reducing body weight and body fat, even with exercise intensity levels as low as 30% VO_2R. Clinicians should be aware that increases in aerobic exercise intensity may be better tolerated after targeted frequencies and durations of training are achieved. Augmentation of daily exercise intensity may also be achieved via the use of occasional sessions of brief higher-intensity exercise.

Cardiorespiratory Energy Expenditure for Body Weight and Body Fat Reduction

Current cardiorespiratory prescription practice for body weight and fat loss is based on the concept of expending a certain volume of work energy in addition to the energy consumed to sustain resting metabolic processes in order to negatively offset the energy consumed in food and liquid nutrients. Unfortunately, the summation of these *estimates* of energy balance does not reliably predict weight change for all patients. In fact, the updated ACSM/AHA (2007) guidelines suggest that exercise produces only modest and relatively variable (i.e., inconsistent) increments in weight loss in excess of the reductions achieved via dietary restriction. Thus, successful exercise prescription is contingent upon the reinforcement of controlled dietary behaviors. Further, the recommended volumes of endurance training to achieve weight loss and prevent weight regain have doubled over the past 10 years and now stand at 60–90 *daily* minutes of moderate-intensity exercise. Clearly, patients exercising at lower levels of intensity face significant challenges.

Lacking still are clear recommendations addressing body composition change in conjunction with weight loss. Whereas some empirical evidence suggests that exercise and controlled diet is more effective than diet alone for helping patients to maintain weight loss and increase muscle weight relative to total body mass, other studies suggest that exercise does not prevent the declines in lean body mass or resting energy expenditure that occur in conjunction with weight loss induced via dietary restriction. Absent also are guidelines addressing whether progressive increments in effort are needed to sustain weight loss as weight loss commences, as is suggested by both theory and clinical practice. Clearly, the complex relationships between energy regulation, body mass, and body composition are yet to be fully understood. While the development of novel methods of manipulating energy balance holds promise (e.g., endocannibinoid receptor blockade), obesity practitioners would be wise to help patients develop systems of self-reward for achieving *consistent health behaviors* in addition to specific energy balance targets, as many patients will not achieve the volumes of physical activity that precipitate a return to normative levels of body mass and composition, even in conjunction with calorie-controlled dietary behaviors.

Resistance Training

Resistance training is designed to increase the size and maximal strength of the large skeletal muscle groups, thereby promoting functional independence across the lifespan. Muscle-strengthening activities also help to reduce cardiovascular stress and certain types of chronic pain and lower the risks for developing, osteoporosis, hypertension, and diabetes. Although resistance training has little direct effect on cardiorespiratory fitness, muscular strength and endurance do facilitate the duration and intensity with which aerobic activities can be performed. As part of a balanced exercise plan, strength training also helps to prevent weight gain and the accumulation of body fat via its influence on energy balance. However, strength training consumes energy at a lower rate than aerobic training, and while it may help to spare the net reduction of muscle mass during weight loss efforts, total resting energy expenditure will decline as weight loss progresses. Hence, resistance training should always be performed in *conjunction* with, rather than at the expense of, cardiorespiratory training when attempting to reduce body mass and body fat.

The intensity of resistance training is difficult to measure, as HR is disproportionate to intensity within this mode of exercise, and the seemingly easy method of counting maximum repetitions (RM) produces highly variable results between individuals and even between muscle groups. Alternatively, intensity may be defined in terms of the progressive recruitment of muscle fiber motor units, with maximum intensity occurring at the point of volitional failure during contraction. So defined, high-intensity strength training can be achieved using inversely varying permutations of the resistance-by-repetition algorithm. Intensity may also be increased by using slower and more controlled movements while maintaining constant muscle tension. All permutations resulting in muscular failure within a concentrated effort produce similar improvements in muscle strength, size, and endurance.[4] Thus, obese patients who are not at risk from exposure to brief but extreme elevations in blood pressure can typically perform resistance training with high intensity, even with low levels of cardiorespiratory fitness. Submaximal training may also facilitate strength development if the overload stimulus surpasses a minimal, but incompletely understood, threshold. The ACSM suggests submaximal termination points corresponding to increased concentric repetition duration, RPE values between 12 and 16, or 1–3 repetitions before muscle failure.

The updated ACSM/AHA (2007) exercise guidelines recommend the performance of 8–10 resistance exercises on 2 or more nonconsecutive days each week targeting the major skeletal muscle groups, using a resistance that allows 8–12 repetitions before volitional fatigue. Progression is achieved by performing increasing volumes of work before failure within the concentrated effort (aka "a set"). Progression may be facilitated by using varied activities to provide more novel stimuli for each specific muscle group, and this process may also improve exercise adherence for some patients. Cross-training also helps to reduce repetitive orthopedic stresses and involves the greatest number of muscle groups. Clinicians should, however, attempt to tailor prescribed activities to the particular interests of each patient, as there is no evidence suggesting differential effectiveness for the varying activities that target any specific muscle group. In addition, most research suggests that single-set strength training regimens are as effective as multiple-set regimens. This creates an opportunity to improve exercise efficiency and potentially long-term adherence[5] for a fair percentage of patients, as the latter method is still commonly practiced at many fitness centers. Finally, exercise prescription should reinforce good form that involves a complete and painless range of motion, a controlled and moderate repetition duration (concentric and eccentric motions of ~ 3 s each), and a normal breathing pattern without breath holding (i.e., exhale during concentric motion, inhale during eccentric motion). Patients engaging in circuit training to simultaneously achieve cardiorespiratory and strength training should be counseled to not exceed a rate of sequential exercises that compromises good form.

Cool Down

A brief cool-down period of approximately 5–15 min helps bodily systems return to normative resting states in a safe manner by facilitating venous blood return, lactic acid removal, and the dissipation of body heat. Cool-down periods are particularly important for patients with cardiovascular disease, as the process also helps to reduce the post-exercise rise in plasma catecholamines that is associated with increased incidence of ventricular dysrhythmias and sudden cardiac death. Cool down is a relatively simple process wherein endurance activities are performed with gradually diminishing intensities.

Safety Concerns for Healthy and At-Risk Populations

Empirical evidence suggests that musculoskeletal injuries do not occur more frequently in physically active populations versus inactive populations, as enhanced physical fitness tends to offset the increased risk for exercise-related injuries. Similarly, moderate-intensity aerobic exercise does not lead to higher rates of sudden cardiac arrest or myocardial infarction in otherwise healthy adults, and aerobic fitness is associated with a 25–50% lower risk of developing cardiovascular disease. Hence, exercise testing and other specialized medical screening procedures are not recommended when prescribing physical activity for low-risk, asymptomatic patients (AHA/ACSM, 2007).

The health risks of physical activity do vary, however, as a function of exercise modality and intensity, as well as the behavioral and physical characteristics of each patient. Therefore, clinical exercise prescription should strive to balance patients' overall health by modifying physical activity targets in response to their changing physical abilities and disabilities. High impact and vigorously performed activities are contraindicated for patients who demonstrate musculoskeletal vulnerabilities or who have cardiovascular, pulmonary, or metabolic disease. In addition, the ACSM recommends that patients with hypertension, diabetes, or at risk for stroke or other medical risks resulting from high blood pressure should avoid high-intensity strength training. These patients should obtain a thorough medical evaluation, including ascertaining possible medication interactions, prior to beginning or significantly increasing their levels of physical activity. Exercise testing and pulse oximetry may be used to set a safe HR range for patients with cardiovascular or pulmonary diseases and those taking medications that alter HR response to exercise, such as β-blockers. Research has demonstrated that these patients can then safely monitor their exercise using RPE and ancillary pain rating scales.

All patients, regardless of health status, should be advised to discontinue exercise and seek medical attention should they experience adverse symptoms other than transient muscle and joint soreness, such as sharp, intense, or persisting pain; significant inflammation; heavy or tight feelings in the chest; irregular heartbeat; breathing difficulties; discontinued or atypical sweating; dizziness; numbness; headache; or nausea. Additionally, patients who have little experience with strength training may benefit from a period of instruction from a certified fitness instructor. Comprehensive information is available from the American Council on Exercise, the National Board of Fitness Examiners, and the American College of Sports Medicine. Obesity providers are encouraged to develop a referral base of instructors who are familiar with the special needs of patients who are medically or physically compromised and those having lower levels of fitness or poor athletic skills.

Considerations for Age, Gender, and Functional Disability

All four modes of exercise can be performed effectively throughout the lifespan, and each is a necessary component of healthy aging. In fact, the most recent AHA/ACSM (2007) exercise guidelines for individuals greater than 65 years of age and those having chronic medical disorders or physical limitations are not substantially different from the guidelines for healthy younger adults. Older patients experience relative improvements in cardiorespiratory fitness and muscle development that are similar to younger patients, although they tend to adapt and progress at slower rates. In order to set appropriate treatment goals, obesity practitioners should also remember that aging is associated with declining $VO_{2\,max}$, muscle strength, and muscle mass, and increasing fat and total body mass. When relevant as a target of treatment, improvements in bone mineral density can be facilitated in older patients via progressive increments in resistance targets during strength training. Useful resources for information about aging and health are provided by the National Institute on Aging and the American Federation for Aging Research.

Relatively few, if any, modifications need to be made to prescribed exercise plans on the basis of gender. On average, men have a higher $VO_{2\,max}$ and more strength than women, due to their larger hearts and more numerous muscle fibers. However, these differences are much smaller when adjusting for relative levels of fat-free body mass, and women respond to endurance and strength training similar to men. Clinicians should be aware that exercise training may produce menstrual irregularities in some women, and women are more susceptible than men to orthopedic injury when performing high-impact, lower-extremity exercise. Pregnancy is of course a condition requiring special exercise considerations that are beyond the scope of this discussion. The interested reader is directed to publications from the American College of Obstetrics and Gynecology.

Case Example

This case example is of a Caucasian male, 61 years of age, receiving primary-care treatment for obesity, cardiovascular disease, Type 2 diabetes, and obstructive sleep apnea. His relevant medications upon starting a hospital-based outpatient behavioral modification program targeting healthy lifestyles were transdermal nitroglycerin 0.4 mg/h, furosemide 60 mg/day, irbesartan 300 mg/day, carvedilol 50 mg/day, aspirin 325 mg/day, atorvastatin 40 mg/day, metformin 2000 mg/day, glipizide 10 mg/day, and pioglitazone 30 mg/day. The patient attended 2 days of intensive education and subsequently received a 60-min behavioral therapy session once per month for 16 months. The patient's initial weight was 316 lb (BMI $= 43$), and his abdominal circumference was 55 in. Weight and behavioral data were collected every 34 days on average (SD $= 4$). Average 30-day trailing caloric intake was 1445 kcal/day (SD $= 50$); average fat, carbohydrate, and protein percentage were 29%

(SD = 2.4%), 45% (SD = 2.5%), and 25% (SD = 1%); and the patient additionally consumed one 12-ounce glass of beer each week. At 16 months, this patient weighed 215 lb (BMI = 29), and he had lost 32% of his starting weight and 18 in. from his waist. Body fat as measured via bioimpedance dropped 3 points in the first 4 months but was not measured thereafter due to the insertion of a cardiac regulatory device.

The patient's baseline levels of physical activity consisted of playing golf twice weekly using a motorized cart and performing light activities of daily living. In the first month, the patient added only light walking as he felt fatigued on his reduced calorie diet in conjunction with poor compliance with his continuous positive airway pressure machine. Over the first 2 months, the patient progressively increased his walking activity as his breathing got easier. After 4 months, the patient was using a bilevel positive airway pressure machine, swimming every other day, and performing light resistance training with dumbbells in addition to his biweekly golf outings and occasional evening walks. Also by this time, his nitroglycerin, pioglitazone, and glipizide dosages had been halved. After 6 months, the patient purchased an elliptical machine to use at home to replace swimming during the winter months. Just shy of 8 months, the patient was diagnosed with an atrial-ventricular block and had immediate surgery to implant a pacemaker. The patient recovered quickly and was able to return to light physical activity in the form of golf at the end of 9 months, at which time he was no longer using pioglitazone. At the end of 12 months, the patient no longer needed his bilevel positive airway pressure machine. At the end of 13 months, the patient no longer used glipizide, and he had added walking stairs to his exercise regimen. At the end of 14 months, the patient began walking the golf courses he played, and his daily aspirin dosage was reduced by one-third. Finally, at the end of 16 months, the patient was walking golf courses 3–5 times each week in addition to various combinations of dumbbell training, walking stairs, and evening walks.

In this case example, the vast majority of the patient's exercise was performed with low but progressing intensity. Incorporation of a variety of aerobic and resistance exercises facilitated adherence to the prescribed exercise plan, and increasing his frequency and duration of exercise within the context of a well-balanced and calorically controlled diet led to weight loss at every one of the patient's follow-up sessions. Interestingly, this patient reports that he was not required to perform exercise-specific cardiac testing to establish a safe maximum HR, even after the insertion of his pacemaker. He was simply advised to exercise with limited exertion, and he was aware of the symptoms of adverse physiological reaction to exercise. This approach was likely influenced by the patient's exceptional adherence to all facets of treatment. Finally, in addition to significant weight loss and reduction in necessary medications, the patient experienced improvements in sleep, mood, and feelings of well-being.

Notes

1. Contrary to ACSM terminology, the author has included body composition only within the physiological components of physical fitness, as it is clearly not a performance-based component, as are the other indices of health-related physical fitness.
2. Two other types of stretching – "dynamic," involving repetitive bouncing movements and "proprioceptive neuromuscular training," involving alternating muscle contraction and relaxation with the assistance of a partner – are not recommended for clinical populations due to their greater risk of muscle strain and injury.
3. Research has shown that initial levels of cardiorespiratory fitness and maximum cardiorespiratory capacity are genetically influenced, with citations as high as 80% for VO_{2max}.

4. Muscle endurance is defined as the number of repetitions to failure at a specific resistance.
5. Resistance training regimens greater than 60 min in duration are associated with higher dropout rates.

Recommended Readings

American College of Sports Medicine. (1995). *ACSM's guidelines for exercise testing and prescription* (7th edn.). Baltimore, Maryland: Williams & Wilkins.

Borg, G. (1985). *An introduction to Borg's RPE-scale*. Ithaca, New York: Movement Publications.

Fletcher, G. F., Balady, G., Blair, S. N., Blumenthal, J., Caspersen, C., Chaitman, B., et al. (1996). Statement on exercise: Benefits and recommendations for physical activity programs for all Americans. A statement for health professionals by the committee on exercise and cardiac rehabilitation of the council on clinical cardiology, American Heart Association. *Circulation, 94*, 857–862.

Kesaniemi, Y.A., Danforth, E.J., Jensen, M.D., Kopelman, P.G., Lefebvre, P., & Reeder, B.A. (2001). Dose-response issues concerning physical activity and health: An evidence-based symposium. *Medicine & Science in Sports & Exercise, 33*(6), S351–S358.

National Institutes of Health. (2004). *Exercise: A guide from the National Institute on Aging and the National Aeronautics and Space Administration* (NIH Publication No. 01-4258). U.S. Department of Health and Human Services, Public Health Service, National Institutes of Health, National Institute on Aging. Retrieved on September 25, 2007, from http://www.nia.nih.gov/HealthInformation/Publications/ExerciseGuide/default.htm

National Institutes of Health. (1998). *Clinical guidelines on the identification, evaluation, and treatment of overweight and obesity in adults: The evidence report* (NIH Publication No. 98-4083). National Heart, Lung, and Blood Institute in cooperation with the National Institute of Diabetes and Digestive and Kidney Diseases. Retrieved on September 25, 2007, from http://www.nhlbi.nih.gov/guidelines/obesity/ob_gdlns.htm

National Institutes of Health Consensus Conference. (1996). Physical activity and cardiovascular health. *Journal of the American Medical Association, 276*, 241–246.

Noble, B.J., & Robertson, R.J. (1996). *Perceived exertion*. Champaign, Illinois: Human Kinetics.

Pate, R.R., Pratt, M., Blair, S.N., Haskell, W.L., Macera, C.A., & Bouchard. et al. (1995). Physical activity and public health: A recommendation from the Centers for Disease Control and Prevention and the American College of Sports Medicine. *Journal of the American Medical Association, 273*, 402–407.

Pollock, M.L., Gaesser, G.A., Butcher, J.D., Després, J.P, Dishman, R.K., Franklin, B.A., et al. (1998). ACSM position stand on the recommended quantity and quality of exercise for developing and maintaining cardiorespiratory and muscular fitness, and flexibility in adults. *Medicine and Science in Sports & Exercise, 30*(6), 975–991.

Saris, W. H. M., Blair, S. N., van Baak, M. A., Eaton, S. B., Davies, P. S. W., Di Pietro, et al. (2003). How much physical activity is enough to prevent unhealthy weight gain? Outcome of the IASO 1st Stock Conference and consensus statement. *Obesity Reviews 4*(2), 101–114.

Scherer, S., & Cassady, S.L. (1999). Rating of perceived exertion: Development and clinical applications for physical therapy exercise testing and prescription. *Cardiopulmonary Physical Therapy Journal. Fall.* http://findarticles.com/p/articles/mi_qa3953/is_199910/ai_n8859094.

U.S. Department of Health and Human Services. (1996). *Physical activity and health: A report of the Surgeon General*. Atlanta, GA: U.S. Department of Health and Human Services, Centers for Disease Control and Prevention, National Center for Chronic Disease Prevention and Health Promotion. Retrieved on August 22, 2007, from http://www.cdc.gov/nccdphp/sgr/contents.htm

Chapter 9
Bariatric Surgery

John C. Linton and Robert B. Shin

Obesity is a costly international public health problem, due to the serious medical co-morbidities associated with it and the financial commitment required for its treatment. Obesity in the United States is increasing at an alarming rate. More than half of the US population is overweight, and of them, half are considered obese. The most common quantification of obesity is the body mass index (BMI), which is the measure of an individual's weight in relation to height and is expressed as the person's weight in kilograms divided by the square of the height in meters. The World Health Organization classifies obesity into three categories: Class I (BMI 30–35), Class II (BMI 35–40), and Class III (BMI>40).

From 1986 to 2000 the number of obese adults in the United States doubled, and the number of extremely obese quadrupled (Sturm, 2003). About a half to two-thirds of Americans are considered either overweight (BMI 25–30) or obese (BMI of 30 or higher). As of 2005, about 15 million Americans had a BMI greater than 35. About half of these fall into Class III, with BMIs exceeding 40, or being more than 100 lb overweight, classifying them as having clinically severe or morbid obesity. While this group includes all races and ages, the majority are women of childbearing age, and they appear to be overrepresented by individuals who are ethnic minorities, impoverished, and poorly educated (Ali, Fuller, Choi, & Wolfe, 2005).

Health Co-morbidities

The National Institutes of Health announced in 1998 that severely obese patients have a 50–100% increased risk of premature death, due primarily to threats from coronary heart disease, hypertension, hyperlipidemia, hypoventilation and sleep apnea, and diabetes. They also suffer high rates of osteoarthritis (Pi-Sunyer, 1993). Their 12-year examination of over 300,000 men and 400,000 women found that mortality rates doubled for men who were 50% above average weight, with a fivefold increase for diabetics and threefold increase in men with digestive tract disease.

In women the mortality rate also doubled, with obese diabetic women showing an eightfold increase in mortality, and tripled in obese women with digestive tract disease. A prospective study in Scandinavia found even moderate obesity was associated with a

J.C. Linton (✉)
Department of Behavioral Medicine & Psychiatry, West Virginia University School of Medicine, Charleston, WV, USA

L.C. James, J.C. Linton (eds.), *Handbook of Obesity Intervention for the Lifespan*, DOI 10.1007/978-0-387-78305-5_10, © Springer Science+Business Media, LLC 2009

dramatic increase in diabetes and amplified as the obesity became more pronounced. Cancer mortality rates are also increased in severely obese females (endometrium, gallbladder, and uterine/cervix) and males (colorectum and prostate) (Sjostrom, 1999). Obesity is now second only to smoking among the top 10 causes of preventable death in the United States (Torquati, Lutfi, & Richards, 2007), and clearly young overweight people die earlier than those with normal weight.

Psychological Quality of Life in Morbid Obesity

The social stigma of being severely obese is well known, with the supposition being that body weight is not regulated physiologically, but instead reflects the obese individual's harmful food habits and psychological needs. In addition to the stigma from society at large, obese patients often feel disrespect from health-care professionals. Many medical offices and hospital facilities are not sensitive to the special requirements of the super obese, for example, their need for oversized or reinforced chairs, accessible rest room facilities, and scales that are calibrated to be capable of weighing them, located in private areas rather than hallways.

Primary-care clinicians can underestimate the connection between obesity and poor self-esteem, which often begins in childhood, and may be set off by abuse. This low self-image becomes hard wired, much like in traumatic stress disorders, and some abuse literature suggests that those who have been exploited become obese to present a less tempting target for future abuse. Even without an abuse history, psychological obstacles for overweight children and adolescents include social stigmatization, teasing by peers, discontent with their bodies, depression, and low self-esteem. Unfortunately, this poor self-image in obese adolescents often remains steady into adulthood (Lowry, Sallinen, & Janicke, 2007).

Others view the super-obese as unhygienic, socially unattractive, less intelligent, self-indulgent, immature, and lacking self-control in many areas of functioning. Because of a negative body image, obese individuals regularly try to avoid public scrutiny, which makes it difficult to put themselves on display to exercise or to engage in recreation in clothing that might reveal their body shape, such as shorts or a bathing suit. Obesity is also linked with a lack of enjoyment of sexual activity, problems with sexual performance, and shunning of sexual encounters (Kolotkin et al., 2006).

Although the literature is somewhat unclear, true psychopathology is also thought to be increased in this population, with higher rates of significant depression, mood shifts, and even suicidality. Those with extreme obesity (BMI > 40) are at even higher risk for depression and diminished quality of life, and the degree of psychopathology appears to be correlated with the extent of obesity. Overall the psychological status of morbidly obese individuals tends to be significantly worse than those with moderate obesity.

Treatment

The epidemic of obesity in the United States has led to a vigorous pursuit of treatments. Because of the disturbing national trends noted above, the Centers for Medicare and Medicaid Services classified obesity as an illness, and this permits providers to receive reimbursement for obesity treatments. Interventions for weight loss can be summarized as those involving lifestyle changes alone, drug therapy, or bariatric surgery (Powell, Calvin, & Calvin, 2007).

As a result of the severity of obesity as a medical problem, NIH convened conferences to address this problem in 1985 and again in 1991. These conferences developed criteria for treating morbid obesity, including medical and surgical solutions. The 1991 conference determined that surgery was the best method for achieving weight loss, maintaining long-term weight loss, and effectively addressing the serious co-morbidities associated with obesity (Ali et al., 2005). Roux-en-Y gastric bypass (RYGB) and vertical banded gastro-plasty (VBG) were seen as the best procedures for weight loss maintenance and addressing medical co-morbidities.

The first surgery to attempt to correct obesity was performed by Dr. Richard Varco at the University of Minnesota in 1953. Early procedures used the jejunoileal bypass, which was later abandoned due to complications from a high degree of malabsorption resulting in malnutrition, diarrhea, and neurological complications (Buchwald & Buchwald, 2002). Since then the field has matured substantially, and bariatric surgical procedures are now extremely popular in the United States and throughout the world, due in part to media coverage and the success of high-profile celebrities, who have lost huge amounts of weight in the public eye.

All physicians should become familiar with bariatric surgical operations, to discover when to refer their patients for this procedure, and how to manage them post-surgically. It is also important that allied health providers who may come in contact with such patients understand the motivation for an individual's seeking bariatric surgery and the demands of their post-operative adjustment.

Types of bariatric surgery can be grouped based on the mechanism through which it is believed that weight loss is achieved. Approximately 85% of bariatric operations performed in the United States are RYGB, followed by laparoscopic adjustable gastric band (LAGB), such as lap band, and biliopancreatic diversion (BPD) with or without duodenal switch (DS). The gastric sleeve operation, originally designed to be a first-stage operation prior to completion of the DS, has gained some attention as a primary bariatric operation, but it is still investigational. VBG is no longer recommended by most reputable bariatric centers in the United States, due to its complications.

The mechanism of surgical weight loss is to either restrict caloric intake by creating a small gastric reservoir (*gastric restrictive procedure*), by introducing malabsorption by bypassing variable length of small intestine (*malabsorptive procedure*), or by *combining both gastric restriction and malabsorption*. By 2003, nearly two-thirds of bariatric operations have been performed laparoscopically since the first laparoscopic gastric bypass and adjustable banding in the early 1990s.

Gastric Restrictive Procedures

These procedures act largely through restriction such as gastric banding (adjustable gastric banding or vertical gastric banding). They work by limiting caloric intake through reducing the size of the gastric reservoir and restricting the outlet, while preserving the GI continuity.

Laparoscopic Adjustable Gastric Banding

Since its introduction in early 1990s, LAGB has become the most commonly performed gastric restrictive procedure and the second most commonly performed bariatric operation worldwide. It has gained significant popularity in the United States since its FDA approval in 2002. The advantage of the LAGB is technical ease, adjustability, and the absence of staple lines or need for the creation of new anastomosis.

In this procedure, a silastic band is placed around the proximal stomach just below the gastroesophageal junction, creating a small gastric pouch approximately 15 ml in volume. The gastric outlet tightness is adjusted by controlling the volume of saline by use of a subcutaneous access port. Achieving appropriate restriction with adjustments is critical for successful weight reduction.

Because the gastric banding procedure does not require the use of staplers, creation of anastomosis, or intestinal bypass, there is no risk of gastrointestinal leaks or malabsorptive complications. Operative mortality and morbidity are reported to be from less than 0.1 to 0.5% by experienced surgeons. This procedure can also be completely reversed. Early postoperative complications include acute obstruction (<1.8%), gastroesophageal perforation (0.4%), early prolapse (0.3%), PE (0.2%), bleeding, port-infection, and open conversion (<1.1%).

Long-term complications from LABG include access port and tubing problems (leak, infection), gastric prolapse (slippage of the band), stomal obstruction, esophageal and gastric pouch dilation, and gastric erosion. Most late complications after LABG can be managed laparoscopically or by a local outpatient procedure. Incidence of port-related complication is around 2–6%. After excluding gastric erosion, port infections are managed by removal of the port and placing the band tubing back into the peritoneal cavity. After complete resolution of local infection and wound healing, the port is replaced at a different site after retrieving the tubing laparoscopically. Replacing the access port and the distal tubing can easily treat a leak. The incidence of esophageal or gastric pouch dilation is less than 6.6%. This is resolved with band deflation.

The incidence of gastric prolapse has reduced significantly as we started to place the gastric bands in the pars flaccida technique (2–3%) rather than the peri gastric approach (10–24%) with minimal dissection. Symptoms of progressive reflux, vomiting, or dysphagia refractory to band deflation are further studied with an upper-gastrointestinal series. A laparoscopic approach is used to reduce the prolapse of the stomach with a band reposition or replacement. The incidence of gastric erosion is less than 2%. With port-site infections or failure of weight loss, laparoscopic removal of the band is recommended.

Weight loss after laparoscopic adjustable band is much more gradual compared with other bariatric procedures. Successful patients can expect to lose 1.5–2 lb/week with proper adjustment to create adequate gastric restriction. Studies have shown that this procedure can result in the loss of about 40–50% of the excess body weight at 2 years, which is significantly less than RYGB or malabsorptive procedures. The need for reoperation, mainly due to lack of weight loss, may be as high as 30% in initial US trials. LAGB requires much more discipline from the patient compared with other bariatric procedures, as well as careful follow-up with appropriate adjustments. If the band is not adequately adjusted, then there will not be proper restriction on the amount of food intake, resulting in inadequate weight loss. Additional reasons for inadequate weight loss after LAGB are as follows:

- Excessive consumption of high-calorie liquids, such as soup, ice-cream, high-fat or sugar shakes, chocolates, or candies
- Excessive snacking between meals
- Poor stress coping mechanisms – stress eating or snacking

Vertical Banded Gastroplasty

Once the most common bariatric procedure in the United States since its introduction in the early 1970s, the number of VBG surgeries has decreased significantly since 1991, despite its relative technical simplicity and low rate of complications. This is mainly due to failure to maintain long-term weight loss secondary to staple line dehiscence and gastric pouch enlargement and significant acid reflux causing severe esophageal irritation.

A small gastric pouch, 15–20 ml in volume, is created with a stapler without division from the rest of the stomach. The gastric outlet is reinforced with a mesh. Operative mortality and morbidity are reported to be about 0.1 and 5% by skilled surgeons. In their meta-analysis, Buchwald, Avidor, and Braunwald (2004) reported an overall excess body weight loss of 68.2%, but most studies report weight loss in the 50–60% range. However, long-term successful weight loss, defined as loss of more than 50% of excess body weight, has been poor, with 38% at 3 years and 30.2% at 10 years.

Malabsorptive Procedures

In these procedures, weight is lost due to malabsorption secondary to increased gastric emptying rates and accelerated intestinal transit times.

Biliopancreatic Diversion or Duodenal Switch

In terms of pure weight reduction and resolution of medical co-morbidities, malabsorptive procedures have produced the best outcome. Biliopancreatic diversion has been routinely performed in Europe since the report by Scopinaro (1991) showing excellent short-term and long-term weight loss of 74% at 2 years and 78% at 14 years. Others have reported 73% excess body weight loss at 51 months after DS.

However, despite superb weight loss outcomes compared with the other bariatric procedures, less than 3% of all bariatric surgeries in the United States have been BPD or DS, mainly due to the significant incidence of side effects such as protein-calorie malnutrition, fat-soluble vitamin deficiencies, severe diarrhea, and osteoporosis. Selection of compliant patients, pre- and postoperative patient education, and close long-term follow-up are mandatory. At our center the DS is considered for patients with super-obesity (BMI greater than 60) or those who have failed previous bariatric operations.

These operations combine malabsorptive intestinal bypass, primarily responsible for weight loss, with restrictive partial gastrectomy. Operative mortality and morbidity are reported to be about 1 and 5%, respectively, by skilled surgeons. Most deaths have been due to pulmonary embolism (PE) (1–2%), myocardial infarction, anastomotic leak (0.1%), and sepsis. Other early complications include gastric perforation, gastric retention, duodenal blowout, anastomotic fistula, pancreatitis, bleeding, and wound complications.

The most common late complications include incisional hernia (18%, but less with a laparoscopic approach) and anastomotic ulcer (6.3–12%). Other possible long-term complications include severe protein-calorie malnutrition up to greater than 15%, with hypoalbuminemia, anemia, edema, asthenia, and alopecia. Also seen are fat-soluble vitamin, iron and folate deficiencies, diarrhea, and osteoporosis due to calcium and vitamin D deficiencies. Careful patient education in lifelong dietary supplements and long-term follow-ups are mandatory.

Combination (Restrictive and Malabsorptive) Procedures

These procedures operate through a combination of malabsorption and restriction. Gastric bypass was first performed in 1966, but there have been many improvements and revisions in the procedure since then.

Roux-en-Y Gastric Bypass

RYGB is the standard bariatric surgical procedure, and approximately 85% of bariatric procedures performed in the United States are the RYGB. This procedure combines both a restrictive element by creating a small gastric pouch (15–25 ml in volume) along the lesser curvature and malabsorptive element by bypassing the duodenum and proximal jejunum. The gastric pouch is stapled off from the rest of the stomach to minimize the occurrence of a gastro-gastric fistula. The remnant stomach maintains its secretion and hormonal functions with no significant physical atrophy. The jejunum is divided 40–50 cm from the ligament of Trietz, and the distal jejunum (Roux limb) is brought up to the gastric pouch. The gastrojejunostomy (gastric outlet) to the Roux limb of the jejunum is created to be approximately 1.2 cm in diameter. This can be performed in hand-sewn or with stapling techniques (linear stapler or end-to-end stapler).

A routine intraoperative leak test for the gastrojejunostomy is done in most centers, such as endoscopic air leak test or methylene blue infusion test. This also creates a dumping syndrome, where the contents of the stomach empty too quickly into the intestines, resulting in diarrhea, nausea, vomiting, weakness, dizziness, and stomach cramping. This unpleasant condition helps the patient avoid foods high in sugar or fat through negative reinforcement. Operative mortality and morbidity are reported to be less than 0.5 and 5% by experienced surgeons. At our center, with experience of more than 1200 laparoscopic RYGB, our mortality is less than 0.2% (30-day mortality), with a 90-day complication rate of less than 2%.

The laparoscopic approach is thought to have a slightly higher rate of intraabdominal complications compared with the open approach, such as gastrointestinal leaks, internal hernia, and gastrojejunal stricture. However, recent studies revealed that in the hands of experienced laparoscopic surgeons, who have undergone a steep learning curve, there was no significant difference in postoperative mortality and morbidity.

Two of the most devastating postoperative complications are gastrointestinal leak and PE. The most common cause of death from RYGB has been PE, with a reported incidence of approximately 0.6%. The reported incidence of gastrointestinal leak is between 1.2 and 4.2%. Our rate of PE is about 0.5%, and gastrointestinal leak is less than 0.2%.

The most important aspect of managing PE is early ambulation after the surgical procedure. The patient is required to ambulate 2 h after extubation. Prophylactic treatments with subcutaneous Lovenox 30 mg BID, starting immediately after the procedure, and pneumatic compression devices are mandatory. Patients are monitored continuously with pulse oximetry and a cardiac monitor. Consideration for prolonged anticoagulation therapy (usually 4 weeks postoperatively) is also recommended for higher risk patients (male, BMI > 50, severe sleep apnea, inability to adequately ambulate, severe diabetes).

Early detection is critical in the management of gastrointestinal leak. Subsequent sepsis, multi-organ failure, and death can be prevented with the intraoperative leak test, routine placement of a drainage tube, and early surgical exploration. Persistent tachycardia is the cardinal sign of the leak, as well as other devastating complications such as PE, bleeding, bowel obstruction, or pneumonia. Persistent tachycardia (heart rate > 120) for more than 4 h, despite aggressive fluid resuscitation, may require urgent surgical exploration. Other signs of possible leak include persistent left shoulder pain, discoloration of drainage fluid, leukocytosis, and persistent hyperglycemia. Routine postoperative radiographic studies are recommended by some centers, but not all. If the leak is detected early, this can be managed laparoscopically with repair and drainage tube placement. If the patient is in sepsis with late detection, surgical placement of a drainage tube without primary repair to control the leak and aggressive nutritional support (via G-tube, J-tube, or TPN) with appropriate antibiotics are recommended.

Other reported early postoperative complications include GI bleeding (about 2%), splenic injury (0.7–2.5%), seroma or superficial wound infection (11.4–14.5%), deep wound infection (3–4.4%), and pneumonia (about 0.14%). Late complications include incisional hernia (4.7–23.9%) that is reported to be more common in the open approach (11% vs. 24%), marginal ulcer (0.2–13.3%), gastric outlet stenosis (3.4–14.6%), small-bowel obstruction (4.7%), and symptomatic gallbladder disease (10–11.4%). With the more popular laparoscopic approach, we are seeing more internal hernia as a cause of small-bowel obstruction or intermittent abdominal pain.

Other long-term complications from RYGB include the dumping syndrome and possible mineral and vitamin deficiencies of iron, folic acid, vitamin B, and calcium. However complications due to mineral and vitamin deficiencies can be minimized or treated effectively with a careful follow-up protocol from bariatric centers and improved patient education and adherence.

Reported expected weight reduction after RYGB is about 65–70% of excess body weight, with maximal weight loss at 2 years postoperatively. Long-term weight loss of 50–60% excess body weight has been documented up to 14 years postoperatively.

Studies report resolution or improvement of the following medical co-morbidities after RYGB:

Glucose intolerance	98.7% resolution
Diabetes mellitus type II	83% resolution
Hypertension	60–73% resolution
Obstructive Sleep Apnea	94.8% resolution or improvement
Hyperlipidemia	96.9% resolution or improvement
GERD	75–85% resolution

Other conditions, such as pseudo-tumor cerebri, urinary stress incontinence and arthropathy, have shown very positive response to RYGB.

Improvement in Co-morbidities by Procedure

A meta-analysis by Buchwald et al. (2004) found that *type 2 diabetes* was resolved in 98.9% of patients who underwent BPD or DS, 83.7% for RYGB, and 47.9% for gastric banding. *Hypertension* was resolved in 81.3% for BPD or DS, 75.4% for RYGB, and 38.4% for gastric banding. *Obstructive sleep apnea* was resolved in 95.2% for BPD or DS, 86.6% for

RYGB, and 94.6% for gastric banding. *Hyperlipidemia* was improved in 99.5% for BPD or DS, 93.6% for RYGB, and 71.1% for gastric banding.

Eligibility Criteria and Patient Selection for Bariatric Surgery

Regarding which patients should be considered for bariatric surgery, anyone who has struggled with morbid obesity or obesity with serious medical co-morbidities can be viewed as a candidate. The patient must be able to understand the necessary postoperative dietary and lifestyle changes.

Potential bariatric surgery patients have been evaluated mostly in retrospective reviews and cohort studies, rather than randomized clinical trials. They have been evaluated for mechanism of weight loss and short-term success, reflecting operative safety and in-hospital morbidity and mortality, and long-term efficacy, reflecting weight loss and maintenance, and postoperative complications.

The 1991 NIH Consensus Development Conference Statement on Gastrointestinal Surgery for Morbid Obesity recommended surgical treatment for patients whose BMI exceeds 40 kg/m^2, or BMI 35 kg/m^2 or more with obesity related co-morbidities, such as diabetes, hypertension, sleep apnea, severe arthropathy, hyperlipidemia, and other cardiopulmonary conditions. An active history of alcohol or substance abuse or uncontrolled psychiatric disease should be screened very carefully.

Psychological Screening

Potential bariatric surgery patients are almost always required to undergo a psychological assessment before acceptance into candidacy for the procedure. These evaluations are typically comprised of a comprehensive structured clinical interview, as well as personality testing or the use of surveys such as the Weight and Lifestyle Inventory (Wadden & Sarwer, 2006). The goal of the appraisal is to report to the bariatric team the unique needs or psychological difficulties a particular patient may be bringing to them. A good evaluation should determine the patients' motivation for surgery and specifically whether it is for example primarily for health enhancement (best), cosmetic benefits (fair), or to save a failing relationship (poor).

Also important is an estimate of patients' cognitive functioning, intelligence, and judgment, their knowledge about the specifics of the procedure, its risks and complications, and a detailed examination of their understanding of what will be required of them after surgery. Understanding their eating patterns and incentive for overeating, such as loneliness, stress reduction, or to be sociable, helps the dietician to better conceptualize potential impediments to their making a lifestyle change. A history of eating disorders, such as binging, nocturnal eating, induced vomiting or laxative abuse to lose weight, and drastic fasting, or the use of bizarre diets should be assessed. Their experience with, motivation for, and obstacles to an exercise regimen is also important for the staff to know.

Assessing other addictions, such as to gambling, alcohol, or drugs, as well as dependence on other foods or beverages that will be contraindicated after surgery will assist the team in gathering a more comprehensive picture of the unique challenges patients might face after this life-altering intervention. It can also be enlightening to examine their networks of social support, as well as any concern or disagreement about their decision for surgery from important people in their lives, who may be in a vital position to enhance or diminish their chances for success after surgery.

Also significant is past psychiatric history and the management and stability of any current psychiatric symptoms. Psychiatric problems are widely recognized as more prevalent in patients who seek bariatric surgery. They are at increased risk for depression, poor quality of life, negative body image, and history of abuse. They also have characteristics similar to those seen in individuals subjected to discrimination and prejudice (Puzziferri, 2005). However, patients who are in psychiatric treatment and stable, and perhaps controlled successfully on psychoactive medications, can be acceptable candidates for surgery.

Generally, accepted reasons for rejection on psychological grounds include severe situational stress, active drug or alcohol abuse, inability to understand or comply with postsurgical guidelines, a clear history of noncompliance with earlier medical care, or untreated psychiatric illness. Sometimes the decision may be to delay the procedure until problems of concern are addressed or the timing is better for the individual. For example, marital other personal or vocational crises will overburden a patient who is also trying to make a radical lifestyle change after surgery.

The Bariatric Team

Once patients are referred to a bariatric center, a multidisciplinary team of a nurse, nutritionist, psychologist or psychiatrist, and surgeon should carefully evaluate them. The weight loss procedure, risks, and the need for long-term follow-up must be emphasized. It is important for patients to have realistic expectations and understand that lifelong dietary and behavioral changes are necessary. Well-informed, motivated, compliant, and supported patients achieve the best long-term success from weight loss procedures. They should be carefully screened and evaluated preoperatively for obesity-related medical co-morbidities, to assess and reduce operative risk factors. Advanced age, previous abdominal procedures, or failed bariatric procedures are not contraindications. Substantial data also support offering weight loss procedures to adolescents, but only after a careful multi-disciplinary evaluation, including family counseling.

Lifetime medical care for postoperative bariatric patients is recommended. In this program, patients are seen at 1 week, 4 weeks, 3 months, 6 months, 9 months, and 12 months after their bariatric operations. After this, we recommend follow-up every 6 months for the next 4 years, then every year for the rest of their lives.

Comprehensive postsurgical follow-ups are critical. Patients need to reestablish healthier but manageable eating behaviors, dietary choices, lifestyle and exercise routines, so it is necessary to provide continuous, consistent and timely support from a dedicated nutritionist, exercise physiologist, and psychologist, as well as from a bariatric surgeon.

Here all patients are also required to participate in nutritional consultations at 4 weeks, 6 months, and 1 year after their bariatric operations. This is necessary to provide adequate nutritional support, since patients experience very significant dietary restrictions. The importance of adequate hydration and the intake of necessary vitamins, minerals, and protein supplementation are emphasized. Weekly classes are also offered to our postsurgical patients from a psychologist, nutritionist, or exercise physiologist, as well as other medical experts.

Matching Patients to Procedures

The decision about which procedure is used is typically made by patient preference. The benefits of RYGB are emphasized in patients with super morbid obesity (BMI greater than 60) and in those with other significant medical co-morbidities (such as severe insulin-dependent diabetes or severe sleep apnea). However, the ultimate decision should come from the patient. Many studies have demonstrated that compliant, committed, and well-educated patients do well from any proven bariatric operation. Weight loss by BPD seems to be most profound and suited to superobese patients. For those at risk for nutritional problems and for whom reversibility of RYGB is unacceptable, banding might be preferred. A sweet eater will fail banding and will need bypass.

Insurance Coverage

Most insurance companies, including Medicare/Medicaid, cover bariatric operations. Most require at least 6 months of medically supervised diet or weight loss attempts prior to any surgical treatment. While this is seen as a justifiable requirement, most individuals who seek bariatric surgery report an extensive history of trying multiple diets and other more conservative ways to lose weight, often since adolescence, and these have failed to stop the progression in weight gain. So this stipulation for an additional period of conservative treatment is questionable, especially when the patient has significant weight-related health problems. This requirement can also eliminate from consideration potentially eligible patients who did not keep or maintain precise medical records.

Further, some insurance plans will not cover preoperative evaluations by a psychologist or a dietician, and this inflicts a financial burden that some patients cannot afford The cost of surgery varies from institution to institution, but many studies have shown that bariatric surgery can be cost-effective in 2–4 years, in comparison with non-operative managements (Safadi, 2005). Unfortunately, some employers may also put a rider in their benefit policies excluding bariatric surgery.

The Bariatric Center of Excellence

Television programs and newspaper articles have reported deadly complications from gastric bypass surgery. So for safety reasons many physicians are reluctant to refer their patients for gastric bypass or lap band. Bariatric operations, especially laparoscopic procedures, do have a very steep learning curve for surgeons to perform. Even with technically less demanding gastric banding, there is always a possibility of having very serious postoperative complications.

In the past many surgeons trying to learn these procedures laparoscopically, some without appropriate training, created damaging outcomes. However, with experience it has been demonstrated that bariatric operations can be safe and effective in treating or improving many medical co-morbidities. Once patients have found surgeons with ample experience and proven safety records, any bariatric operation can be performed safely.

For these reasons, referring patients to Bariatric Centers of Excellence with documented experience, safety, and proper patient education, and postoperative follow-ups is very important to maximize patient safety, minimize long-term complications such as mineral and vitamin deficiencies, and ensure the best long-term weight loss maintenance. Physicians should first consider referring their patients to Centers of Excellence approved by the American Society of Metabolic and Bariatric Surgeons (ASMBS) or the American College of Surgeons (ACS).

A Center of Excellence (COE) in Bariatric Surgery will be able to provide comprehensive care with a multidisciplinary staff. Our COE has a nurse practitioner, nurse coordinator, dietitians, a psychologist, an exercise physiologist, and administrative staff to manage the insurance approval process. The most important aspect of the COE is patient safety. Proper patient education, patient selection, and reduction of preoperative risk factors are critical objectives that must be met from the surgeon's office.

The hospital must provide an appropriate environment for obese patients (suitable chairs, rooms, doors, showers, and toilets) and equipment such as special instruments for surgeons. Also necessary are well-trained intraoperative assistants, OR staff and anesthesiologists, availability of needed medical specialties and facilities, and a dedicated nursing staff. Long-term follow-up is crucial to promote patient adherence, to prevent vitamin, mineral, and nutritional deficiencies and to produce lasting weight loss. Multidisciplinary staff counsel the patient in dietary, behavioral, emotional, lifestyle, exercise, and medical issues on regular basis.

Continued staff education is another important feature of the Bariatric COE. This includes, for example, obesity sensitivity training, dealing with postoperative complications, new technology, patient care improvements, and inter-departmental communication.

Many studies show that it takes 100–125 bariatric cases for a surgeon to master the steep learning curve. A significantly higher rate of morbidity and mortality rates are found in the earlier part of surgeon's experience, that is, a surgeon who has performed less than 50 cases per year or a center that performs less than 120 cases per year. Thus, in order to be designated as a COE, a surgeon must perform more than 50 bariatric cases per year, with at least 120 total cases in a facility where at least 120 bariatric cases are performed annually.

Future Developments

Like any surgical field, achieving minimal invasiveness in procedures has been aspirational. Efforts to achieve this is have included performing procedures through natural orifices, such as doing bariatric operations with endo-luminal approaches through the mouth with endoscopic instrumentation.

There is also strong interest in expanding this field into metabolic surgery, to eventually cure metabolic syndrome or type II diabetes in non-obese populations. There has been animal research as well as some smaller studies from outside of the United States to support this direction of inquiry.

Insurance companies will likely have no option but to cover these procedures in the future. However, the question is how accessible these operations will be. Not only is bariatric surgery the most effective treatment to lose excess weight, but also this is one of the most effective medical treatments to resolve type II diabetes, sleep apnea, GERD, hypertension, and other very serious medical co-morbidities. All patients will continue to need sound preoperative work-ups, meticulous surgical technique, prompt response to complications, and sustained postoperative follow-up. The greatest success will come with patients who scrupulously comply with a 12–18 month exacting and habitual monitoring protocol.

Demand for these procedures should be steady due to the worsening trend toward obesity in the United States. Further, as we can demonstrate less postoperative morbidities and mortalities with more experience, or new less-invasive modalities, public demand may well accelerate.

Bariatric surgery is not the cure for obesity. But it is the most effective tool available to help lose weight and among the most gratifying procedures general surgeons perform, with dramatic weight loss, management of co-morbidities, and patient satisfaction higher than for any other general surgical procedure.

Unfortunately, many patients, frustrated from many failed weight loss attempts, view a bariatric operation as an "easy way out" or a foolproof last option. Both patients and some surgical teams are under the impression that undergoing a bariatric surgical procedure will lead to a controlled, inevitable weight loss. But this is the only "behavioral surgery." In order to produce long-term success, making proper behavioral, dietary, lifestyle, and exercise modifications are crucial. Many patients regain their weight after significant initial weight loss after RYGB or do not lose adequate amount of weight after gastric banding, due to failure to make these necessary postoperative changes.

In sum, there is no doubt that obesity-related diseases dramatically resolve or improve after bariatric surgery. No other medical or surgical intervention simultaneously treats as many disease processes as does bariatric surgery (Brethauer, Chand, & Schauer, 2006). Carefully screened patients treated by skilled, experienced bariatric surgeons in a COE offer many patients their best hope for life enhancement, and in some cases survival.

References

Ali, M.R., Fuller, W.D., Choi, M.P., & Wolfe, B. M. (2005). Bariatric surgical outcomes. *Surgical Clinics of North America, 85*, 835–852.

Brethauer, S., Chand, B., & Schauer, P.R. (2006). Risks and benefits of bariatric surgery: Current evidence. *Cleveland Clinic Journal of Medicine, 73* (11), 993–1007.

Buchwald, H., & Buchwald, J. (2002). Evolution of operative procedures for the management of morbid obesity 1950–2000. *Obesity Surgery, 12*, 705–717.

Buchwald, H., Avidor, Y., & Braunwald, E. (2004), Bariatric surgery: As systematic review and meta-analysis. *JAMA, 292*, 14, 1724–1737.

Kolotkin, R.L., Binks, M., Crosby, R.D., Ostbye, T., Gress, R.E., & Adams, T.D. (2006). Obesity and sexual quality of life. *Obesity, 14*, 3, 472–479.

Lowry, K.W., Sallinen, B.J., & Janicke, D.M. (2007). The effects of weight management programs on self-esteem in pediatric overweight populations. *Journal of Pediatric Psychology, 32*, 1179–1193.

Pi-Sunyer, F.X. (1993). Medical hazards of obesity. *Annals of Internal Medicine, 119*, 655–60.

Powell, L.H., Calvin, J.E., & Calvin, J.E. Jr. (2007). Effective obesity treatments. *American Psychologist, 62* (3), 234–246.

Puzziferri, N. (2005). Psychologic issues in bariatric surgery-the surgeon's perspective. *Surgical Clinics of North America, 85*, 741–755.

Safadi, B.Y. (2005). Trends in insurance coverage for bariatric surgery and the impact of evidence based reviews. *Surgical Clinics of North America, 85*, 665–680.

Scopinaro, N. (1991). Why the operation I prefer is biliopancreatic diversion. *Obesity Surgery, 1*, September, 307–309.

Sjostrom, C.D. (1999). Reduction in incidence of diabetes, hypertension and lipid disturbances after intentional weight loss induced by bariatric surgery: The SOS intervention study. *Obesity Research, 7* (5), 477–84.

Sturm, R. (2003). Increases in clinically severe obesity n the United States. *Archives of Internal Medicine, 163*, 2146–48.

Torquati, A., Lutfi, R.E., & Richards, W.O. (2007). Predictors of early quality of life improvement after laparoscopic gastric bypass surgery. *The American Journal of Surgery, 193*, 471–75.

Wadden, T.A., & Sarwer, D.B. (2006). Behavioral assessment of candidates for bariatric surgery: A patient centered approach. *Obesity, 14* (Suppl), March, 53–62.

Part III
Treatment Resources for Providers

Books, NIH and Journal Helpful References

Aronne, L. J. (1997). Weigh Less, Live Longer. Published by Wiley.

Brownell, K. (2004). The LEARN Program for Weight Management. Published by the LEARN Education enter.

Brethauer, S., Chand, B., & Schauer, P.R. (2006). Risks and benefits of bariatric surgery: Current evidence. *Cleveland Clinic Journal of Medicine, 73*(11), 993–1007.

Buchwald, H., & Buchwald, J. (2002). Evolution of operative procedures for the management of morbid obesity 1950–2000. *Obesity Surgery, 12*, 705–717.

Buchwald, H., Avidor, Y., & Braunwald, E. (2004). Bariatric surgery: As systematic review and meta-analysis. *JAMA, 292*, 14, 1724–1737.

Earles, J.E., Kerr, B., James, L.C., & Folen, R.A. (2007). Clinical effectiveness of the LEAN Program: A military healthy lifestyle program. *Journal of Clinical Psychology In Medical Settings.*

Earles, J., James, L.C., Folen, R.A., & Verschell, M. (2001). *Incorporating behavioral telehealth in the treatment of obesity.* A Poster Presented at The American Psychological Convention, August San Francisco.

Epstein, L. H. (1996). Family-based interventions for obese children. *International Journal of Obesity*, 20(Supp. 1), S14–S21.

Epstein, L. H., Valoski, A., Wing, R. R., & McCurley, J. (1994). Ten-year outcomes of behavioral family based treatment for childhood. *Health Psychology*, 13, 373–383.

Fairburn, C.G., & Brownell, K.D. (2005). *Eating disorders and obesity*(2nd ed.). New York: Guildford Press.

Fletcher, G.F., Balady, G., Blair, S.N., Blumenthal, J., Caspersen, C., Chaitman, B., et al. (1996). Statement on exercise: Benefits and recommendations for physical activity programs for all Americans. A statement for health professionals by the committee on exercise and cardiac rehabilitation of the council on clinical cardiology, American Heart Association. *Circulation, 94*, 857–862.

Kesaniemi, Y.A., Danforth, E.J., Jensen, M.D., Kopelman, P.G., Lefebvre, P., & Reeder, B.A. (2001). Dose-response issues concerning physical activity and health: An evidence-based symposium. *Medicine & Science in Sports & Exercise, 33*(6), S351–S358.

Kolotkin, R.L., Binks, M., Crosby, R.D., Ostbye, T., Gress, R.E. & Adams, T.D. (2006). Obesity and sexual quality of life. *Obesity, 14*, 3, 472–479.

Kotz, C.M., Billington, C.J., & Levine, A.S. (1999). Obesity and aging. *Clinics in Geriatric Medicine, 15*(2), 391–412.

Lowry, K.W., Sallinen, B.J., & Janicke, D.M. (2007). The effects of weight management programs on self-esteem in pediatric overweight populations. *Journal of Pediatric Psychology, 32*, 1179–1195.

McTigue, K.M., Hess, R., & Ziouras, J. (2006). Obesity in older adults: A systematic review f the evidence for diagnosis and treatment. *Obesity, 14*(9), 1483–1497.

National Center for Health Statistics. (2004). Health, United States, 2004, with Chartbook on Trends in the Health of Americans. Hyattsville, MD: U.S. Department of Health and Human Services, Centers for Disease Control and Prevention.

National Institutes of Health Consensus Conference. (1996). Physical activity and cardiovascular health. *Journal of the American Medical Association, 276*, 241–246.

Noble, B.J., & Robertson, R.J. (1996). *Perceived exertion.* Champaign, Illinois: Human Kinetics.

Pate, R.R., Pratt, M., Blair, S.N., Haskell, W.L., Macera, C.A., Bouchard, C., et al. (1995). Physical activity and public health: A recommendation from the Centers for Disease Control and Prevention and the American College of Sports Medicine. *Journal of the American Medical Association, 273,* 402–407.

Pi-Sunyer, F.X. (1993). Medical hazards of obesity. *Annals of Internal Medicine, 119,* 655–660.

Pollock, M.L., Gaesser, G.A., Butcher, J.D., Després, J.P, Dishman, R.K., Franklin, B.A., et al. (1998). ACSM position stand on the recommended quantity and quality of exercise for developing and maintaining cardiorespiratory and muscular fitness, and flexibility in adults. *Medicine and Science in Sports & Exercise, 30*(6), 975–991.

Powell, L.H., Calvin, J.E., & Calvin, J.E. Jr. (2007). Effective obesity treatments. *American Psychologist, 62*(3), 234–246.

Sezginsoy, B., Ross, K., Wright, J.E., & Bernard, M.A. (2004). Obesity in the elderly: Survival of the fit or fat. *Journal of the Oklahoma State Medical Association, 97*(10), 437–442.

Villareal, D.T., Apovian, C.M., Kushner, R.F., & Klein, S. (2005). Obesity in older adults: Technical review and position statement of the American Society for Nutrition and NAASO, The Obesity Society. *Obesity Research, 13*(11), 1849–1863.

Wadden, T. A., & Stunkard, A. J. (2002). *Handbook of obesity treatment.* New York: Guilford.

Wadden, T.A., & Sarwer, D.B. (2006). Behavioral assessment of candidates for bariatric surgery: A patient centered approach. *Obesity, 14*(Suppl), March, 53–62.

Wing, R.R. (1997). Behavioral approaches to the treatment of obesity. In G. Bray, C. Bouchard, & P.T. James (Eds.).

Web-Based Resources

National Institutes of Health. (2004). *Exercise: A guide from the National Institute on Aging and the National Aeronautics and Space Administration* (NIH Publication No. 01-4258). U.S. Department of Health and Human Services, Public Health Service, National Institutes of Health, National Institute on Aging. Retrieved on September 25, 2007, from http://www.nia.nih.gov/HealthInformation/Publications/ExerciseGuide/default.htm

National Institutes of Health. (1998). *Clinical guidelines on the identification, evaluation, and treatment of overweight and obesity in adults: The evidence report* (NIH Publication No. 98-4083). National Heart, Lung, and Blood Institute in cooperation with the National Institute of Diabetes and Digestive and Kidney Diseases. Retrieved on September 25, 2007, from http://www.nhlbi.nih.gov/guidelines/obesity/ob_gdlns.htm

Exercise: A Guide from the National Institutes on Aging: A publication to encourage exercise among older adults, promoting safety and motivation. Web address: http://www.nia.nih.gov/HealthInformation/Publications/ExerciseGuide/

Physical Activity for Everyone: Are There Special Recommendations for Older Adults: A comprehensive website by the Centers for Disease Control and Prevention on exercise recommendations for older adults, strength training programs for older adults, and motivational and goal-setting tools. http://www.cdc.gov/nccdphp/dnpa/physical/recommendations/older_adults.htm

NIH Senior Health: An interactive website by the National Institutes on Aging to assist older adults when beginning an exercise program. Web address: http://nihseniorhealth.$gov/exercise/toc.html

The Calorie King for counting calories. A helpful reference for assisting patients to determine the amount of calories and fat in their meals. WWW.CalorieKIng.Com

Index

Note: The letters '*f*' and '*t*' following the locators refer to figures and tables respectively

Printed in the United States of America